Poultry Practice

The *In Practice* Handbooks Series

Series Editor: Edward Boden

Past and present members of *In Practice* Editorial Board

Titles in print:
Feline Practice
Canine Practice
Equine Practice
Bovine Practice
Sheep and Goat Practice
Swine Practice
Small Animal Practice
Poultry Practice
Equine Practice 2

The *In Practice* Handbooks

Poultry
Practice

Edited by E. Boden
Executive Editor, *In Practice*

Baillière Tindall

LONDON   PHILADELPHIA   TORONTO   SYDNEY   TOKYO

<u>Baillière Tindall</u>   24–28 Oval Road
W. B. Saunders   London NW1 7DX

The Curtis Centre
Independence Square West
Philadelphia, PA 19106–3399, USA

55 Horner Avenue
Toronto, Ontario, M8Z 4X6, Canada

Harcourt Brace Jovanovich Group
(Australia) Pty Ltd
30–52 Smidmore Street
Marrickville
NSW 2204, Australia

Harcourt Brace Jovanovich Japan Inc
Ichibancho Central Building
22–1 Ichibancho
Chiyoda-ku, Tokyo 102, Japan

Typeset by Photo·graphics, Honiton, Devon
Printed and bound in Hong Kong by Dah Hua Printing Press Co., Ltd.

A catalogue record for this book is available from
the British Library

√ISBN 0–7020–1687–X

Contents

Contributors   vii

Foreword   ix

1. **Health and welfare of animals in modern husbandry systems—poultry:** M. Pattison   1
   Introduction. Preventive medicine. Respiratory signs. Diarrhoea. Drop in egg production. Poor "quality" chicks/poults. Stunting syndrome. Leg problems. Miscellaneous. Common conditions seen in other types of stock. Laboratory support. Welfare

2. **Common conditions resulting in poultry carcase condemnation:** C. Stuart   17
   Introduction. Septicaemias. Air sacculitis. Aspergillosis. Hydropericardium. Egg peritonitis. Neoplasms. Emaciation. Salphingitis. Breast blisters. Skin lesions. Major damage. Overscald. Poor bleeding. Liver lesions. Salmonellosis. "Green leg". Contamination

3. **Respiratory conditions of the fowl:** F. T. W. Jordan   31
   Introduction. Clinical signs and lesions. Epidemiology. Diagnosis. Control

4. **Parasitic conditions in poultry 1: protozoal**   59
    diseases: A. J. Trees
    Introduction. Coccidiosis in chickens. Coccidiosis
    in turkeys. Histomoniasis. Cryptosporidium.
    Other protozoa

5. **Parasitic conditions in poultry 2: helminths and**   73
    arthropods: A. J. Trees and W. Beesley
    Introduction. Nematodes of the respiratory tract.
    Intestinal nematodes. Other intestinal nematodes.
    Cestodes. Control of helminthiases. External
    parasites of poultry

6. **Vaccination regimes for poultry:** D. L. Haxby   87
    Introduction. Basic considerations. Vaccination
    programmes

7. **Common diseases in turkeys reared for the**   95
    Christmas market: I. MacPherson
    Introduction. Arrival of poults. Important diseases
    in the first two weeks of life. Diseases of the post
    brooding period—enteric. Respiratory diseases of
    the post brooding period. Skeletal disorders

8. **Diseases of game birds:** S. Lister   115
    Introduction. General management. Disease
    problems. Brooder problems (0–2 weeks). Rearing
    problems (2–8 weeks). Release and adult
    problems. Conclusions

    Index   131

Contributors

W. Beesley University of Liverpool, School of Tropical Medicine, Department of Veterinary Parasitology, Pembroke Place, Liverpool L3 5QA, UK

D. L. Haxby Candant House, Main Street, Upton, Newark, Nottinghamshire NG23 5ST, UK

F. T. W. Jordan University Veterinary Field Station, Leahurst, Neston, South Wirral, Merseyside L64 7TE, UK

S. A. Lister McLintock House, 21 Chapelfield Road, Norwich, Norfolk NR2 1RR, UK

I. MacPherson Former Director, Hoechst UK Ltd, Animal Health Division, UK

M. Pattison Mortimer Cottage, Westmore, Mansel Lacy, Hereford, Hereford and Worcester HR4 7HN, UK

C. Stuart (deceased) Former President of the British Veterinary Poultry Association

A. J. Trees University of Liverpool, School of Tropical Medicine, Department of Veterinary Parasitology, Pembroke Place, Liverpool L3 5QA, UK

Foreword

In Practice was started in 1979 as a clinical supplement to *The Veterinary Record*. Its carefully chosen, highly illustrated articles specially commissioned from leaders in their field were aimed specifically at the practitioner. In the form of "opinionated reviews", they have proved extremely popular with experienced veterinarians and students alike. The editorial board, chaired for the first 10 years by Professor James Armour, was particularly concerned to emphasize differential diagnosis.

In response to consistent demand, articles from *In Practice*, updated and revised by the authors, are now published in convenient handbook form. Each book deals with a particular species or group of related animals.

E. Boden

CHAPTER 1

Health and Welfare of Animals in Modern Husbandry Systems— Poultry

MARK PATTISON

INTRODUCTION

The approach to clinical problems in poultry inevitably differs a little from other species, but basic principles of medicine and pathology, applied with a degree of background knowledge of the "normal", should allow the clinician to tackle most problems.

Often in large units problems are of suboptimal production, caused not by classical disease alone but by a subtle combination of management, nutrition and disease factors. The veterinarian is uniquely qualified to tackle these problems and should not be deterred from them.

The breeding companies issue management guides, which show the performance that is expected of their stock. For example, broilers would be expected to achieve a weight of 2 kg at 44 days for males and at 49 days for females at a feed conversion of 2.10. Egg layers might achieve 270 eggs for a laying period of 52 weeks. Turkey growth now is exceptional, with males having a potential to reach 13 kg at 20 weeks, females approximately 4 kg at 10 weeks.

PREVENTIVE MEDICINE

The most significant contribution to poultry health can be made through the discipline of preventive medicine. The clinician should consider advice on the subjects of vaccination programmes, husbandry, nutrition, record keeping and hygiene.

Vaccination programmes are required for breeders and commercial layers, which have a longer life span than broilers or fattening turkeys. Vaccines are of two types: those consisting of live, attenuated or avirulent strains of virus that lend themselves to methods of mass administration by drinking water or aerosol spray; and inactivated vaccines consisting of killed virus and adjuvant, which must be administered individually by injection.

A separate account of vaccination regimes for poultry is given by Haxby (1985) and should be read in conjunction with this paper (see p. 87).

Good husbandry and stockmanship are the most important aspects of poultry farming. The concepts of tender loving care and attention to detail on the farm often make the difference between occurrence or absence of disease. The number of birds on a site and whether it is single- or multi-age are important factors. In general, there are likely to be more problems if there are more than 20 000 breeders or 200 000 broilers on one site.

Siting of rearing houses near to laying houses, as often occurs for egg layer-type birds, means that the site is never empty and this can cause problems. For example, live vaccines used for the rearing birds can infect the birds in lay causing a reaction and drop in egg production. The longer the houses can remain empty the better, but in practice broiler houses are never empty for more than a few days. Depopulation of sites between flocks is always to be aimed for.

A study of accurate records on the farm can enable the clinician to form an impression of the problem, before even examining the birds. A typical broiler record chart is shown in Fig. 1.1.

A farm hygiene programme should recommend cleaning with a power hose, using detergent and disinfectant followed by formaldehyde fumigation. Also the exclusion of wild birds

Age (days)	Mortality Dead	Culls	Feed deliveries	Remarks	Water consumption
1					
2					
3					
4					
5					
6					
7					
8					
9					
.					
.					
.					
60					

Fig. 1.1
A typical broiler record chart.

from poultry houses and limitations on visitors to the site are most important.

The clinician will rarely be asked to make a diagnosis on single birds so it is important to consider the signs shown by the majority of the flock. Ensure birds received for post mortem examination are typical of the flock problem and not "culls" representing normal flock attrition.

As disease now is often complicated by management/ environment factors, it is useful to consider differential diagnosis under groups of clinical signs.

RESPIRATORY SIGNS

Ventilation may be the most important determining factor. So often bad air exchange in the building produces areas of stale air. This in turn leads to ammonia build up and paralysis of cilia with excess mucus seretion in the respiratory tract. An ideal situation is then created for viral or bacterial infection.

There are several viral infections which may occur in broilers.

INFECTIOUS BRONCHITIS

Infectious bronchitis is the most common viral disease. There is an acute tracheitis with increased mucus and inflammatory exudate in the trachea. Commonly, secondary *Escherichia coli* infection becomes established producing pneumonia, air sacculitis and pericarditis. There are many serotypes of infectious bronchitis virus, which makes control by the one type of available vaccine difficult. The only licensed vaccines for infectious bronchitis in the UK are made from the Massachusetts strain of virus. There is now ample evidence of infection with other variant strains of infectious bronchitis virus and the importance of these is currently being investigated.

INFECTIOUS LARYNGOTRACHEITIS

Infectious laryngotracheitis is endemic in certain areas of the country and fowl pox in the respiratory form may closely resemble infectious laryngotracheitis. Both can produce diphtheritic lesions in the trachea. These diseases can be distinguished and confirmed by virus isolation and tracheal histology.

NEWCASTLE DISEASE

Newcastle disease should always be considered in the differential diagnosis of respiratory signs. Diagnosis is based on virus isolation and serology taking into consideration any history of vaccination. Newcastle disease is notifiable and suspicions must be reported to the Ministry of Agriculture divisional veterinary officer.

TURKEY RHINOTRACHEITIS

Turkey rhinotracheitis is a respiratory disease characterized by sudden onset and high morbidity. Birds may be affected at any age and mortality can vary from 1 per cent to over 30 per cent in contiguous groups on the same site.

The initial signs are submaxillary oedema and coughing, followed by a frothy ocular discharge and a sticky exudate from the nares, which is followed by distension of the infraorbital sinuses. The fluid in the sinuses is at first clear and mucoid but subsequently caseous. High mortality in a flock is caused by secondary *E. coli* infection, although the disease itself is thought to be viral in origin. Scattered bacteria have been isolated from early cases including species of *Klebsiella, Bordetella, Moraxella, Staphylococcus, Streptococcus, Proteus* and *Alcaligenes faecalis*.The latter is a mild respiratory pathogen in its own right.

Treatment of respiratory disease is aimed at control of secondary infection. Antibiotics are usually administered in the drinking water: amoxycillin, trimethoprim and furaltodone are the most useful. Sensitivity tests for *E. coli* are helpful in determining a course of treatment. Sometimes a longer course of in feed medication is necessary.

DIARRHOEA

Diarrhoea is a feature of many different situations not always caused by disease. It may have been missed in a deep litter house containing large numbers of birds and the first noticeable feature is that the litter has become very wet. This always seems to happen suddenly, "overnight".

In cases of wet litter, reasons other than disease should be considered first. These include environmental effects resulting from poor ventilation, condensation and drinker spillage. Feed effects can be caused by excess sodium chloride in the ration or an imbalance between excess sodium and potassium. Excess protein, indigestible carbohydrate or the use of poor quality fats can also cause abnormal faeces. For example, baby chicks cannot digest saturated animal fat, such as that in tallow, and ingestion of too much of this type of product produces a black sticky excretion. The quality of drinking water must also be tested, both bacteriologically and for any abnormal chemical constituents.

Coccidiosis is the most likely disease to consider if the stock are replacement breeders or pullets. Broilers are less likely to succumb as a high level of coccidiostat can be fed throughout their short lives. Necrotic enteritis caused by clostridial infection may be a sequel to some forms of coccidial infection, e.g. *Eimeria brunetti,* or may be seen in uncomplicated form. There are now known to be a number of viruses such as rotavirus and "small round" virus that can cause diarrhoea in broilers but their true significance is not known. The ones known to be important are Newcastle disease virus and the adenovirus that causes haemorrhagic enteritis in turkeys.

Records of water consumption are extremely useful as a general indicator of flock health and it is recommended that poultry houses are fitted with water meters.

DROP IN EGG PRODUCTION (Table 1.1)

A drop in egg production is an extremely common reason for the veterinarian being called.

The quality of egg shells may give some clues to the cause of the drop. Abnormal numbers of soft shells are seen in the disease egg drop syndrome, caused by an adenovirus which may be vertically or horizontally spread. Abnormal shapes with excess deposits of calcium may be caused by infectious bronchitis (Fig. 1.2).

Table 1.1 Factors causing a drop in egg production.

Water consumption Failure of the water supply or failure to drink will cause a precipitous drop in egg production.
Feed consumption The wrong type of feed may have been delivered or the wrong formulation given. Poultry farmers are advised to keep samples of each feed delivery, properly labelled, for future reference.
Ventilation This should be satisfactory.
Lighting programme If the birds are on a fixed day length light pattern of 17 hours, an accidental alteration of the time clock can have disastrous results.

The presence of these two conditions can be determined by serology using the haemagglutination inhibition test on paired serum samples, one taken at the onset of the problem and one taken two weeks later. Blood samples should also be tested for Newcastle disease virus. In 1984 a different strain of paramyxovirus type 1 was recognized, which was antigenically distinct from Newcastle disease virus. This virus is carried by pigeons and causes a drop in egg production in layers and breeders.

Epidemic tremor may also cause drops in production in laying stock without other clinical signs. Records must therefore be checked to see if vaccination for this desease was carried out.

Paramyxovirus 3 infection of breeder turkeys seems to be more widespread now, leading to a drop in egg production, with white shelled eggs (Fig. 1.3). Turkey rhinotracheitis infection causes very severe drops in egg production, although birds make a quick recovery and return to normal in about three weeks. Post mortem examinations should be conducted if mortality is excessive and also the physical condition of the birds checked to see if a moult has started. Never forget that pilferage can be the hardest cause of egg loss to diagnose!

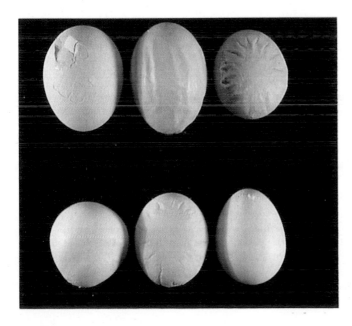

Fig. 1.2
Abnormal shells
typical of infectious
bronchitis infection.

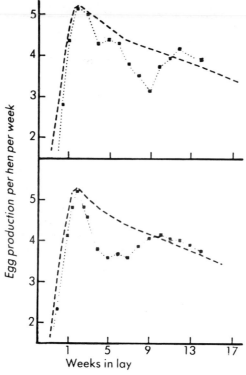

Fig. 1.3
Egg production curve seen in
paramyxovirus 3 infection in laying turkeys.
— — — —, Expected egg production;
■...■..., actual egg production. From
Alexander *et al.*, 1983.

POOR "QUALITY" CHICKS/POULTS

The national average mortality in broiler flocks is 5 per cent, of which up to 2 per cent may be lost in the first two weeks. The most usual reason is yolk sac infection, which may be a sign of poor hatching egg or hatchery hygiene.

Baby chick nephropathy occurs during the first week of life and causes heavy mortality. Birds may die shortly after hatching. The kidneys are swollen and urates are usually deposited on the viscera and in the joints (visceral gout). Chilling or overheating during transport or in the early brooding period causes chicks to die from dehydration or starvation as they may not start to feed. These chicks remain very small. At post mortem examination the gall bladder is distended, the pectoral musculature is very thin and the liver is pale.

STUNTING SYNDROME

A rising mortality during the second week often heralds the onset of stunting syndrome. Affected chicks are small in size and often show retention of chick down where feathers should be growing. There is noticeable abdominal distension caused by dilation of the intestines, which contain large quantities of undigested food.

Lesions are rather variable; there is often a pale, fibrosed pancreas, with sometimes proventricular swelling, thymic atrophy and lesions of rickets in the skeleton. The disease is transmissible and several candidate viruses are being investigated. It appears to be more common in progeny from young breeder flocks and can become endemic on certain sites. A good standard of clean-out and disinfection followed by formaldehyde fumigation appears to reduce the severity of the condition in following flocks.

LEG PROBLEMS

Leg disorders in various forms often account for about 15 per cent of mortality through culling in a typical broiler flock. Dyschondroplasia is common in both broilers and turkeys and may be seen in rapidly growing birds without leg deformity. The lesion consists of a mass of abnormal cartilage, detected by splitting the bone, which extends from the growth plate into the metaphysis. It is most commonly seen in the proximal tibiotarsus (Fig. 1.4) and, if the lesion is large, the cortical bone is weakened resulting in tilting of the proximal end of the bone which may fracture. The condition is more common in males. Affected birds are usually in good condition and the leg often shows a varus deformity.

Valgus deformity ("twisted leg") where the leg bends outwards at the hock joint is also common. The lesion is generally the result of lateral tilting of the distal tibiotarsal condyles, which may eventually separate from the bone. In turkeys the lower third of the distal tibiotarsus may rotate laterally producing a similar valgus deformity. This is a true rotation of the shaft; in most cases only one leg is affected.

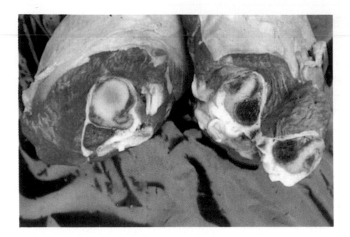

Fig. 1.4
Dyschondroplasia
affecting proximal
tibiotarsus.

Lame broilers with infected hock joints are often seen and these are usually dehydrated and in poor condition. Viral arthritis with tenosynovitis is less commonly seen in the UK than in some other countries. It may result in rupture of the gastrocnemius tendon with associated haemorrhage into surrounding tissues (Fig. 1.5).

If, after post mortem examination, no obvious cause of lameness can be found, the spinal column should always be split to check for the presence of spondylolisthesis ("kinky back"). This condition is caused by downward rotation of the sixth thoracic vertebral body which results in compression of the spinal cord. Affected birds squat back on their hocks and cannot stand. Only broilers are affected.

MISCELLANEOUS

There are two other common conditions occurring in broilers which should be mentioned. Sudden death syndrome ("acute heart failure", "flip over") is seen in broilers from the end of the first week onwards. Birds are found on their backs and the principal post mortem finding is severe pulmonary congestion and oedema. Birds are always in good condition. The cause is unknown and the subject of current research. Ascites and congestive heart failure are seen in most flocks

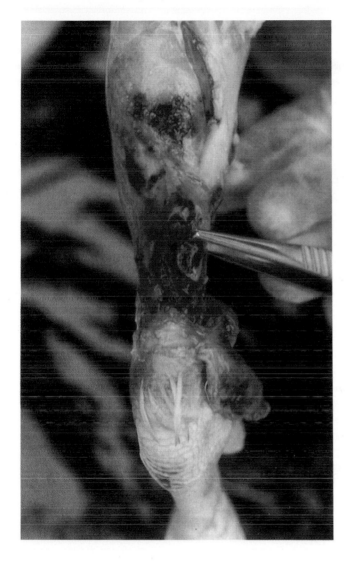

Fig. 1.5
Rupture of
gastrocnemius
tendon following
tenosynovitis.

at a low incidence, but occasionally they flare up and cause flock problems. There is severe passive venous congestion with dilation of the right side of the heart. Often the ascitic fluid is semi-clotted and the musculature shows a deep red colour.

COMMON CONDITIONS SEEN IN OTHER TYPES OF STOCK

BROILER BREEDERS

Broiler breeders are reared on feed restriction from about two to 18 weeks to avoid them becoming too fat for laying. They are therefore under considerable stress, especially at about 12 weeks of age. At this time, staphylococcal infection of the hock joint is an important condition and can cause loss through culling. Treatment with broad spectrum antibiotics is sometimes effective, but must be started early and continued for two or three weeks. This hock condition can be almost eliminated by floor feeding without a trough (Dutchman type) feeder, on which the birds appear to damage themselves. Traumatic injury, often not visible, seems to set off the staphylococcal infection.

Coccidiosis can be troublesome causing mortality and unevenness in broiler breeders during the rearing stage. It can be difficult with a restricted feeding programme to ensure that the birds receive sufficient coccidiostat to prevent disease. The intake of drug must be low enough to ensure that coccidial multiplication occurs and so the birds develop immunity.

An increasing amount of egg peritonitis is being seen in this type of bird at the onset of lay. The cause is unknown.

Breeders should be routinely treated with piperazine twice during rearing to remove any ascaris infection. Capillaria infestation is rare but should always be considered if flocks are not performing well.

Pasteurella multocida infection is sometimes seen, usually in the chronic form causing swollen wattles (Fig. 1.6).

TURKEY BREEDERS

Generally turkey breeders are very healthy. They are, however, susceptible to *P. multocida* infection which can cause high mortality.

The broiler coccidiostats, salinomycin and narasin, are extremely toxic for adult turkeys and their involvement should be considered in the differential diagnosis of sudden death (Fig. 1.7). Before death, birds are seen to pant with wings outstretched and the head tipped forward.

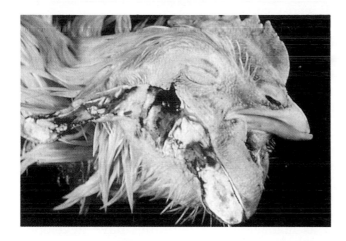

Fig. 1.6
Chronic *Pasteurella multocida* infection in wattles of broiler breeder.

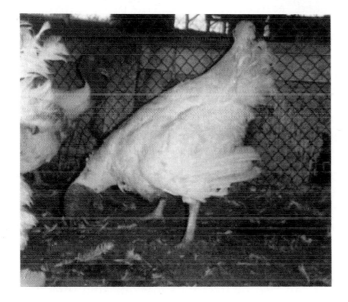

Fig. 1.7
Ionophore poisoning in adult turkey.

COMMERCIAL LAYERS

Commercial layers usually have a low mortality in rearing. In lay, most deaths appear to be caused by prolapse, egg peritonitis, fatty livers, urolithiasis and sometimes tumours such as lymphoid leukosis or Marek's disease. These tumours can be differentiated by histology.

COMMERCIAL TURKEYS

Common conditions diagnosed in commercial turkeys include haemorrhagic enteritis, pasteurellosis and aspergillus infection. There is also a condition called cardiohepatic syndrome, in which poults under three weeks of age are found dead. There is dilation of the right side of the heart with ascites, pale liver and generalized venous congestion. The cause is unknown.

ALL TYPES OF STOCK

Cannibalism can be a problem in all types of stock but is now rarely seen as management techniques have developed to prevent this happening. Broiler breeders are usually "precision debeaked" at five days of age. This process involves removing the tip only of the upper mandible.

Turkey breeders are treated similarly at around three weeks of age, though a little more of the upper beak is removed. If pecking starts, lights are dimmed and wounds can be sprayed with an antibiotic aerosol.

LABORATORY SUPPORT

Poultry practice requires the services of a laboratory, the most important facilities being for bacteriology and serology. The average practice laboratory should be able to carry out mycoplasma serology, using the rapid plate test. (Breeding stock are now sold free from *Mycoplasma gallisepticum, M. synoviae,* and *M. meleagridis.*) They should be monitored once or twice in lay to ensure continued freedom. Monitoring of commercial layers can also be useful as mycoplasma infection in these birds may be the trigger for other virus infections, which can affect egg production.

Many laboratories now carry out haemagglutination inhibition tests for Newcastle disease, infectious bronchitis and egg drop syndrome and gel diffusion tests for gumboro and adenovirus. The haemagglutination inhibition test is useful for monitoring field infection and, or, efficiency of vaccination. Also, post mortem facilities are essential.

WELFARE

Many practitioners carry out official veterinary surgeon (OVS) duties for poultry slaughter plants and will become more involved in welfare duties as time goes on. There is some controversy concerning stunning voltages and the use of lethal stunning may become more common as there seems to be no effect on efficiency of bleed out. From the welfare standpoint, lethal stunning would be preferable.

The OVS duties should also take the practitioner on to the farm from time to time to see birds being caught and loaded. There is an interesting new development called a broiler harvester, rather like a combine harvester, which is now having trials to see if broilers can be mechanically caught. If successful it should improve considerably on "hand" catching which inevitably causes stress and damage to birds with resultant downgrading.

Welfare of poultry in transit is another important aspect. In general, it can be said that the standards that contribute to good welfare also help factory profits, so all points of view are in accord.

Stocking densities for broilers and turkeys are used as guidelines in welfare codes, as a set figure is convenient to work to. Clearly there are maximum limits, but high densities of stocking under conditions of good management may be satisfactory, whereas the same stocking level in poorer conditions may be totally inappropriate.

Recently a small but well defined market has emerged for free-range eggs. This represents the view of a section of the population who do not like birds to be kept in cages. Thus poultry arks in fields are not entirely a thing of the past. However, good management of a cage system for layers makes better economic sense and this in turn takes due consideration of the birds' welfare and efficient disease control.

The Farm Animal Welfare Council, set up in 1979, is keeping under review the welfare of all farm animals, but its work is particularly appropriate to poultry. Codes of welfare initially submitted to ministers in 1982 are continually being evolved through consultation with interested parties and this must be to the benefit of the poultry industry and the consumer.

REFERENCES AND FURTHER READING

Alexander, D. J., Pattison, M. & Macpherson, I. (1983) *Avian Pathology* **12,** 469.

Gordon, R. S. & Jordan, F. T. W. (1982) *Poultry Diseases,* 2nd edn. Eastbourne, Baillière Tindall.

Haxby, D. L. (1985) *Veterinary Record* Supplement *In Practice* **7,** 182.

Randall, C. J. (1985) *Colour Atlas of Diseases of the Domestic Fowl and Turkey.* London, Wolfe Medical.

CHAPTER 2

Common Conditions Resulting in Poultry Carcase Condemnation

CLIFF STUART

INTRODUCTION

Since Poultry Meat Hygiene Regulations 1976 (amended 1979) became fully operational on 15 August 1979, poultry meat may, with a few exceptions, only be sold if it has been subjected to an ante mortem and post mortem inspection, has been hygienically prepared in licensed poultry processing plants, packed, stored and transported under hygienic conditions. All the foregoing must be supervised by an official veterinary surgeon (OVS). Local authorities are responsible to the Minister of Agriculture, Fisheries and Food for the implementation of the regulations. Approximately 100 poultry processing plants require an OVS. Over 250 veterinary surgeons have privately taken a course in poultry meat hygiene run jointly by the British Veterinary Association and the Ministry of Agriculture. Many are fulfilling the duties of an OVS on a part time basis from their practice, a few have taken full time employment with a local authority. All are helped by separately trained poultry meat inspectors.

Carcases are detained by the OVS helped by his team of poultry meat inspectors. They are voluntarily surrendered for condemnation by the processing plant management. If the latter does not agree with the detention the OVS can take the carcases to a magistrate who will decide on evidence presented whether they should be condemned or allowed to go as fit for human consumption.

United States Department of Agriculture returns for 1977 show that 1.23 per cent of all carcases inspected were condemned. The species breakdown of all birds inspected was: 1.07 per cent broilers; 1.44 per cent young turkeys; 2.03 per cent ducks; 3.60 per cent old turkeys; 3.81 per cent old hens. In all the species the two main causes for condemnation were septicaemia and air sacculitis with tumours replacing the latter in old hens.

There are no comparable figures for Great Britain as the Poultry Meat Hygiene Regulations have only been operative since August 1979. However, a recent survey instigated by the British Veterinary Association of those poultry processing plants under the control of an official veterinary surgeon indicates that the level of condemnations in those plants is, if anything, below those in America. Occasional individual flocks, however, fall well outside these figures.

The same USDA returns show that apart from the poundage of poultry meat condemned as whole carcases—231 083 000 lb weight—there was in addition 128 427 000 lb weight of poultry meat condemned as parts of carcases. Comparative figures for Great Britain are not available.

SEPTICAEMIAS

Septicaemias may be acute as in the case of pasteurellosis, erysipelas, salmonellosis, staphylococcosis and most commonly, *Escherichia coli* infections, or produce chronic lesions as seen mainly with *E. coli* infections.

The acute forms, which occur in a small number of cases, show most of the signs of septicaemic carcases typified by the fevered carcase with hyperaemic muscle that appears more reddy-brown than usual, widely distributed petechial haemorrhages, especially in the heart fat and mesenteries (Fig. 2.1), and swollen often enlarged liver and spleen. In less acute cases, small yellow foci of necrotic tissue may be found in the liver.

Most carcases showing these acute forms will be removed at the whole bird inspection point. It is unlikely that one

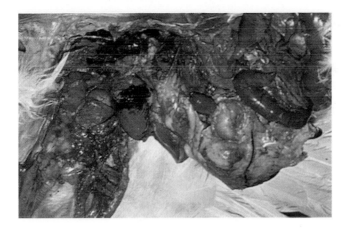

Fig. 2.1
Erysipelas:
haemorrhages on
heart fat and
petechial
haemorrhages on
mesentery.

could differentiate between the different causal agents without resort to laboratory procedures to isolate and identify each agent. The carcases must be detained.

The more chronic lesions in chickens are seen as an extensive serofibrinous pericarditis and perihepatitis, are usually due to *E. coli* infection (Fig. 2.2), but on rare occasions salmonella may be involved. Many carcases with these lesions will show no external signs, others will be emaciated. In some cases this is complicated by concurrent mycoplasma infections when an air sacculitis and/or pneumonia will be present. It is impossible to tell if the causal organisms are still present in the musculature without laboratory examination of each carcase.

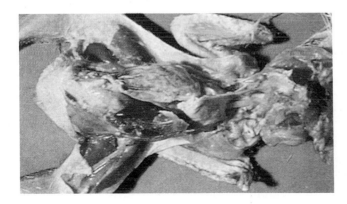

Fig. 2.2
E. coli "septicaemia"
showing as
serofibrinous
pericarditis and
perihepatitis.

If any are still present then the danger to human health, the possible lack of rigor mortis development and the associated reduced lactic acid muscle content resulting in "tough meat", are good reasons to retain the carcases. Unfortunately there are no lymph nodes in poultry that the official veterinary surgeon or poultry meat inspector can use to help him with his judgement of the carcase.

These chronic lesions are less extensive in ducks and rarely seen in turkeys.

AIR SACCULITIS

In broilers air sacculitis is rarely seen without associated *E. coli* lesions of perihepatitis and pericarditis. A viral infection or a factor of bad management in the house will also be involved.

In turkeys it is a disease entity in itself frequently associated with mycoplasma infections and some birds in the affected flock may show swollen infraorbital sinuses. On occasions a viral infection such as Newcastle disease, influenza A or ornithosis may have precipitated the clinical symptoms. However, the aetiology of all cases has not been determined. The extent of the lesions vary from a slight cloudiness of the air sacs with little serous exudate, to completely opaque thickened air sacs containing large amounts of serous exudate (Fig. 2.3). In extreme cases a peritonitis develops. As the

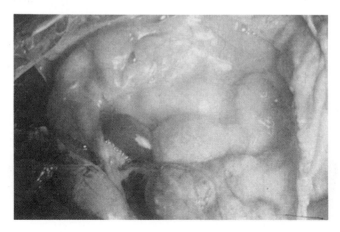

Fig. 2.3
Air sacculitis in a turkey: thickened air sacs full of viscous fluid and core of aspirated material.

condition becomes more chronic the exudate becomes consolidated; the air sacs will contain different sizes of white consolidated material varying from small plaques to large masses that form a complete cast of the air sac. This cheesey material frequently contains *Aspergillus fumigatus* hyphae that can be demonstrated in a laboratory.

In reaching a judgement on carcases with air sacculitis the extent of the condition and its effect upon the whole carcase should be considered. The judgement must essentially depend upon a visual assessment by the OVS/PMI.

When the air sacculitis is associated with a septicaemia or emaciated case, the whole carcase should be retained. In less extensive involvement which show no systemic changes but involvement of the clavicular air sac, the meat should be stripped from the carcase. In the chronic cases the carcase may be passed provided all the air sacs and the contents are removed.

ASPERGILLOSIS

Lesions of aspergillosis are sometimes seen in the air sacs and lungs of large turkeys and ducks. These consist of white plaques of consolidated material surrounding a centre of the greenish blue fructating bodies of the fungus. The Poultry Meat Hygiene Regulations 1976 require that these carcases are totally rejected.

HYDROPERICARDIUM

Cases of hydropericardium which are quite common in broilers should not be confused with those of *E. coli* pericarditis. In the former the pericardial fluid can be quite excessive and the pericardial sac white and thickened, but there will be no endocardial/pericardial adhesions. Only the heart need be retained.

EGG PERITONITIS

This is one of the main conditions seen in end of lay hens, ducks and turkeys. The whole of the abdominal viscera are surrounded by yolk material causing a peritonitis which, in most cases seen in the processing plant, will be of a chronic nature resulting in extensive adhesions of the intestines (Fig. 2.4). Many of these have an offensive odour. The carcase should be retained. In some cases localized lesions occur without any offensive odours. These carcases may be salvaged after removal and retention of the viscera.

NEOPLASMS

Neoplasms are seen in all types of poultry but are most commonly seen in the old hen. There are many different types of tumours. Most of them belong to four classifications: the leucosis group (Fig. 2.5), Marek's disease, diffuse carcinomas involving the pancreas, the ovary, the mesentery and serosal surface of the intestines, and hepatic and renal carcinoma, which are all malignant and require carcase detention.

Benign tumours in individual organs also occur and only require local trimming. Unfortunately, it is frequently

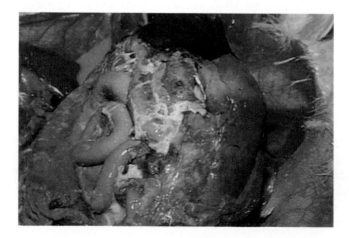

Fig. 2.4
Egg peritonitis: a peritonitis leading to adhesions between the viscera.

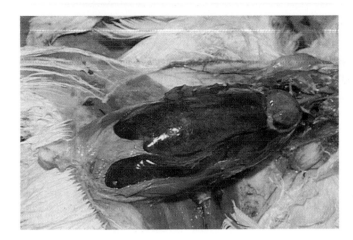

Fig. 2.5
Lymphoid leucosis of
chicken (greatly
enlarged view).

impossible to differentiate between some benign and some malignant neoplasms without resort to histological examinations. If there is any doubt the carcase is retained.

EMACIATION

Emaciation is one of the main reasons for detaining carcases at the whole bird inspection point. In this condition the musculature especially over the sternum and the fatty tissues regresses. Anaemia and ascites may also be present. Causes vary from starvation brought about by any locomotory disorder, or management fault, to birds recovering from a disease outbreak or succumbing to a chronic infection or parasitism.

SALPHINGITIS

Chronic lesions of salphingitis are frequently found in ducks and occasionally in the broiler. These consist of a hard whitish cheesy centre of the immature oviduct. Provided the carcase is normal, and it usually is, stripping out and retention of the diseased organ is all that is required.

BREAST BLISTERS

Breast blisters are often a problem in large chickens and turkeys (Fig 2.6). They may be due to a disease—*Mycoplasma synoviae* infection—in which case some joints may also be affected. Other cases are due to some skeletal disorder or management fault—over-crowding, under-ventilating, etc.—that causes the birds to spend more time on their breasts. The blister will vary in size from that of a small plum to that of a large orange. Uncomplicated cases contain a clear weak tea-like fluid. In some the blister becomes infected by secondary bacterial invaders—*E. coli*, staphylococci, in which case it contains pus. Some of these ulcerate and discharge.

Provided the carcase as a whole is normal, only the blister and any affected surrounding area needs to be trimmed. Areas of loose skin are often found over the sternum. Many of these do not contain any underlying blister and can therefore be ignored.

Small breast blisters should not be confused with infected feather follicles that occur along the side of the breast. These swellings may be quite fibrous or contain pus. They are localized lesions and are trimmed accordingly.

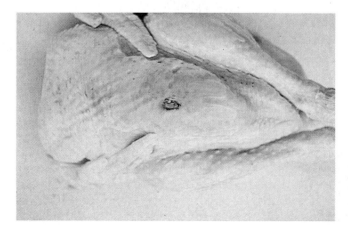

Fig. 2.6
Large ulcerative
breast blister
requiring trimming.

SKIN LESIONS

These may be as a result of a disease or injury on the farm, or due to damage during loading or unloading, or machine damage after slaughter.

Diseases that cause skin lesions in poultry, that are likely to be seen at the processing plant, are rare in Great Britain.

The skin form of Marek's disease produces swollen, whitish nodular, feather follicles (Fig. 2.7) that coalesce in later stages of the disease. They are particularly noticeable along the large feather tracts of the neck, legs and breast areas. One may also see in some birds a white discoloration of the iris and irregular pupil. Others will show internal lesions and swollen nerves, or tumours in the gonads, liver, heart, lungs or musculature. All such carcases are totally unfit for human consumption.

Skin damage caused by birds scratching each other's backs when they climb over each other either due to panic, lack of food, or overcrowding in the houses, can be very extensive. The abrasions become infected and cause the birds condition to deteriorate into emaciation. In others they may be restricted to small areas that will require trimming.

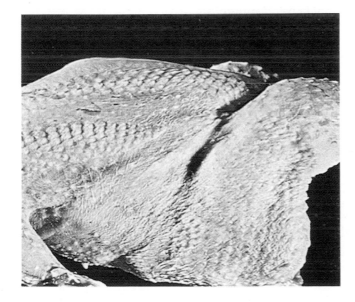

Fig. 2.7
Marek's disease lesion in the feather follicles. A rare condition in the United Kingdom.

MAJOR DAMAGE

Wings may be broken in the fattening house when birds fly about and hit the feeders, etc. These fractures heal in some cases with large callus formation. In others the skin is broken and an infected lesion develops. The latter requires trimming under the Poultry Meat Hygiene Regulations. The former will probably be trimmed by the quality controller of the plant as undesirable in the finished product.

During catching, loading and unloading, wings and legs may be broken or dislocated due to rough handling of the birds. Both result in extensive haemorrhage. Similarly, bruising occurs and may be quite severe. Affected areas should be trimmed from the carcases. It should be noted that blood does seep a considerable distance between layers of muscle and this needs to be exposed. Small lentil-sized haemorrhages are usually ignored. The age of a bruise can be estimated by its colour. There are more precise biochemical tests available.

Ninety per cent of bruises seen in the processing plant occur between 0 and 12 hours before slaughter (May, Hamdy, *WPSA Journal*, **22**, 316) (see Table 2.1).

After slaughter breakages and dislocation of bones do occur due to machine damage in which case they are not

Table 2.1 Gross morphological colour changes in bruises of live broilers as related to time after bruising.

Age of bruise	External appearance at 70°F environment	External appearance at 86°F environment
Control	Normal	Normal
2 min	Red	Red
12 hours	Diffused dark red-purple	Diffused red-purple
24 hours	Diffused light green-purple	Diffused light green-purple
36 hours	Yellow-green-purple	Diffused green-purple
48 hours	Yellow-green (orange)	Dark green
72 hours	Yellow-orange	Almost normal
96 hours	Slight yellow	Normal
120 hours	Normal	Normal

Colours given are those evident on live birds. After death all young bruises revert to a dark red-purple.

accompanied by haemorrhage. Quite extensive skin damage may also occur due to badly designed or adjusted plucking machines.

OVERSCALD

Birds that spend too much time in the scald tank will become slightly cooked—overscald. This usually occurs due to a break in the line or to poor adjustment of the scald temperature and line speed. The skin of affected carcase feels slimy to touch and slips from the underlying meat which is much whiter than usual. If this cooking of the musculature extends deep into the muscles the skin and affected muscle should be trimmed and retained.

POOR BLEEDING

Inadequate bleeding of the carcase is another reason for retention of the whole carcase. This occurs if the birds are septicaemic or die in the stunning process or do not have their necks cut correctly after stunning. The latter occurs with both manual and automatic systems.

LIVER LESIONS

Detention of the liver is required where lesions of blackhead (histomonas) are present in turkeys and chickens (Fig. 2.8). The carcase if satisfactory in all other aspects is fit for human consumption. The same judgement appertains where chronic lesions of *Catena bacterium* (*Avian Diseases* **12**, 417, **16**, 808) occur in the turkey, with extensive fibrosis of the livers in turkeys and ducks and severe dark green discoloration of livers of all species (Fig. 2.9). There is a tremendous variation in the normal red coloration of livers influenced by the fat content. These are fit for human consumption.

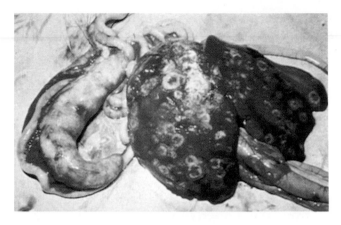

Fig. 2.8
Lesion of blackhead
(histomoniasis) in the
caeca and liver of a
turkey.

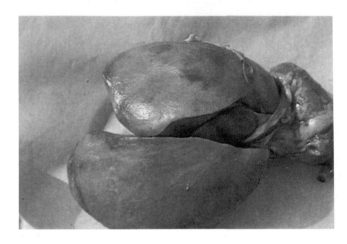

Fig. 2.9
Fibrosis of turkey
liver: the green
coloration is due to
interference with the
bile system.

SALMONELLOSIS

Very little has been said in this article about salmonellosis. It is unlikely that any lesions due to the majority of salmonella serotypes will be found in the processing plants. However, occasionally a serofibrinous pericarditis and perihepatitis indistinguishable from that due to *E. coli* and small necrotic foci in the liver, heart and caeca can be found in broilers, young ducks and turkeys as a result of salmonellosis. The species specific salmonella of poultry will produce detectable lesions, as one would expect. *Salmonella pullorum*, which is not thought to be present in commercial poultry in the country will produce abscesses in the heart, gizzard, pancreas and abnormal angular and irregular shaped ova in the adult. *S. gallinarum*, now fortunately quite rare, will produce small necrotic foci in the livers that show a greenish brown sheen on exposure to the air and abnormal ova.

The catching crates, equipment in the processing plant and carcases become contaminated with salmonella that may be present in the faeces of the birds. Cross contamination of carcases will occur from all these items. This highlights the extreme importance of all efforts to reduce faecal contamination of the carcases, in plant hygiene during the day and end of day clean up procedures.

"GREEN LEG"

This is not a gangrenous condition. There is a total or partial rupture of the gastrocnemius tendon approximately $\frac{3}{4}$ inch proximal to the tibiotarsal-tarsometatarsal joint, which tears the associated blood vessels. The aetiology is confused but probably involves an interrelationship between breed, nutrition, management and the virus of viral arthritis. The green discoloration is due to degradation products of haemoglobin. The affected leg requires trimming and detention.

CONTAMINATION

Contamination and discoloration of the skin with faecal matter or bile necessitates the area to be trimmed. One must not forget the possibilities of other contaminants such as grease from the equipment, denatured rubber marks from the plucker fingers and disinfectants.

Carcases that fall into the feather sluices or the evisceration troughs will be grossly contaminated and these are retained as unfit for human consumption. Carcases that fall on to the floor are fit for human consumption provided that they are washed at once and that they have not been irreversibly contaminated by some foreign material such as grease or disinfectant.

It has been impossible to mention every possible condition that one may see in a poultry processing plant; only the most common ones have been briefly discussed.

These and other conditions fall within those laid down in Schedule 6 of the Poultry Meat Hygiene Regulations as "indications of unfitness for human consumption":

(a) Death resulting from a cause other than slaughter
(b) General contamination
(c) Major lesions and ecchymosis
(d) Abnormal smell, colour, taste
(e) Putrefaction
(f) Abnormal consistency
(g) Cachexia
(h) Oedema
(i) Ascites
(j) Jaundice
(k) Infectious disease
(l) Aspergillosis
(m) Toxoplasmosis
(n) Extensive subcutaneous or muscular parasitism
(o) Malignant or multiple tumours
(p) Avian leukosis complex
(q) Marek's disease
(r) Poisoning

REFERENCES AND FURTHER READING

Bremner, A. S. (1977) *Poultry Meat Hygiene and Inspection*. London, Bailliere Tindall.
Poultry Meat Hygiene Regulations (1976, as amended 1979). London, HMSO.
US Department of Agriculture. Poultry Meat Inspection Regulations.

CHAPTER 3

Respiratory Conditions of the Fowl

FRANK JORDAN

INTRODUCTION

Respiratory conditions of the fowl may be defined as those diseases in which clinical signs and/or gross lesions of the respiratory tract occur with or without lesions in other organs and tissues. An understanding of their epidemiology and methods of diagnosis are a logical prerequisite for control.

Some pathogens directly affecting the respiratory tract of the fowl are given in Table 3.1.

CLINICAL SIGNS AND LESIONS

Clinical examinations of domestic poultry have never attained the sophistication often practised in mammals and abnormal respiratory signs are generally recognized by simple visual and auditory examination.

Table 3.1 Some pathogens directly affecting
the respiratory tract of the fowl.

Viruses
  Newcastle disease (ND)
  Infectious bronchitis (IB)
  Infectious laryngotracheitis (ILT)
  Fowl pox
  Influenza A
  Adenovirus*
  Reovirus*

Bacteria
  Pasteurella multocida
  Haemophilus paragallinarum (*gallinarum*)
  *Escherichia coli**

Mycoplasma
  *Mycoplasma gallisepticum**
  *Mycoplasma synoviae**

Fungi
  Aspergillus fumigatus

Parasites
  Syngamus trachea

It is important to appreciate that multiple
infections occur in which more than one
respiratory pathogen acts concomitantly to
cause disease of the respiratory system.
* Mainly involved in respiratory disease of
multiple aetiology.

NASAL EXUDATE

Nasal exudate frequently accompanies diseases involving
the nasal passages and turbinate bones. It is most copious
and consistently present in such infections as *Haemophilus
paragallinarum* (*H. gallinarum*), causing fowl coryza and *Pasteurella multocida* (fowl cholera). Clear and watery at first, it later
becomes turbid, tenacious and mucoid. In this form it often
dries on the margins of the nostrils to form a dry exudate.

Nasal discharge may also occur in Newcastle disease, avian
infectious bronchitis (IB), infectious laryngotracheitis (ILT),
influenza A, vitamin A deficiency and in mixed infections
but it is inconsistent in appearance, and is rarely as copious
as in the diseases mentioned above.

CONJUNCTIVITIS

Frothy conjunctivitis in which the exudate collects at the anterior canthus is seen frequently in infections with *Haemophilus paragallinarum, Pasteurella multocida* and, occasionally, in Newcastle disease, infectious bronchitis and infectious laryngotracheitis; also on exposure to gaseous ammonia such as occurs with damp litter and inadequate ventilation.

INFRAORBITAL SINUSITIS

The infraorbital sinuses connect directly with the floor of the nasal passages and disease of one or both is manifest by swelling. This results from thickening of the walls and accumulation of mucous exudate. The mucus is at first clear and watery and later tenacious and only rarely becomes inspissated; the condition usually regresses. It may occur sporadically in any of the common respiratory diseases but is most evident in coryza (*H. paragallinarum*) and cholera (*P. multocida*) and mild swelling may accompany *Mycoplasma gallisepticum* infection and influenza A virus infection (Figs 3.1 and 3.2).

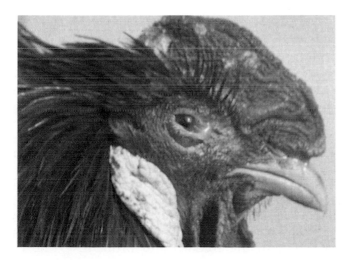

Fig. 3.1
Mild coryza with exudate from the eyes and nares.

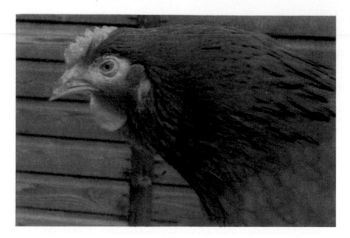

Fig. 3.2
Periorbital swelling.

RÂLES, COUGHING, SNEEZING AND DYSPNOEA

Râles, coughing, sneezing and dyspnoea are indications of some impediment to normal respiration or irritation of the airways and are invariably accompanied by lesions of the larynx, trachea, syrinx or primary bronchi. Exudate is usually present and in mild cases may consist of little more than normal amounts of mucus; in others it may be copious and in some conditions such as infectious laryngotracheitis (ILT) involve sloughed mucosa. In ILT there may be haemorrhage and caseous exudate, sometimes extending the whole length of the trachea. Caseous exudate is sometimes seen in young chickens affected with IB and, rarely, in fowl pox, when it occurs in the region of the larynx (Fig. 3.3).

Râles may be moist or dry and vary with the severity of the disease. In very mild cases they are almost imperceptible and in a flock may not be readily appreciated above the other sounds. The presence of râles is best heard under conditions of darkness when other sounds are muted. Almost all diseases which give rise to an impediment or to exudate in the trachea and bronchi are associated with the above clinical signs. These include the viruses, bacteria and mycoplasma listed, also *Syngamus trachea* and excess ammonia in the environment. *Aspergillus fumigatus* causes dyspnoea but without râles.

Dyspnoea is usually associated with considerable impediment to air movement in the trachea and bronchi. While it

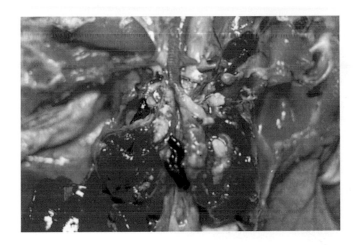

Fig. 3.3
Caseous exudate in
the lower trachea,
primary bronchi and
lungs.

might result from almost any infection, it is most common in
ILT particularly when caseous plugs obstruct the trachea.

Conditions which occur rarely but which can cause coughing
and dyspnoea include vitamin A deficiency with hyperkera-
tosis of the tracheal mucosa, foreign body obstruction such
as a food pellet, and tumours of the trachea. Dyspnoea may
also occasionally occur in Marek's disease when the vagus
and, or intercostal nerves are involved.

LUNG LESIONS (Fig. 3.4)

Congestion of one or both lungs is associated with a
number of the common respiratory diseases but oedema with
consolidation is a frequent feature of *P. multocida* infection.
Caseous lesions in the lung are found in *Salmonella pullorum*
and in some other salmonella infections of young chicks,
tuberculosis of mature birds and *A. fumigatus* infection of
fowls of any age but usually of brooding stock. Petechiae on
the surface of the lungs occur in many acute conditions and
may be particularly marked in severe fowl cholera. Tumours
of the lung are relatively rare but may be seen in the acute
(visceral) form of Marek's disease and leukosis and other
tumours.

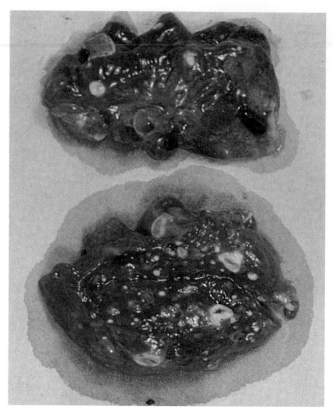

Fig. 3.4
Lesions of
aspergillosis in the
lungs.

AIR SAC LESIONS

The air sac walls are normally transparent but in respiratory disease affecting the air sacs they become increasingly opaque, blood vessels become congested and, if the condition persists, they become oedematous and coated with caseous exudate. In advanced cases there may be caseous casts causing distension of the air sacs, particularly the abdominal, thoracic and interclavicular air sacs. Thickening of the air sac walls may occur with any chronic respiratory disease affecting the lower respiratory tract and is frequently associated with infections involving more than one pathogen (multiple infections). (See *Escherichia coli, Mycoplasma gallisepticum* and *Mycoplasma synoviae*.)

EPIDEMIOLOGY (Fig. 3.5)

Epidemiology may be defined as the study of all the factors associated with disease production in the individual or flock or herd and associated with the transmission of disease. The factors essential for the production of a particular disease are referred to as primary causal factors while others which may predispose to the production or severity of disease or may be ameliorating or preventive in their effect are referred to as influencing or secondary factors.

The severity of disease is influenced by the nature of primary and influencing factors. For disease caused by inanimate primary factors the epidemiology is relatively

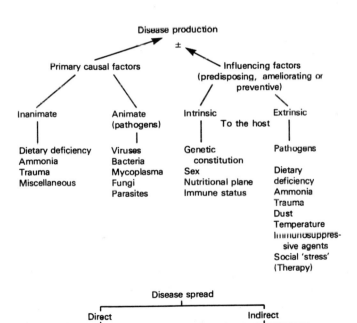

Influencing factors — varieties of host species, stocking density, movement of infected birds, survival of the causal agent within the host and in the environment, movement of fomites and other carriers of infection, numbers of pathogens.

Fig. 3.5 Epidemiology of respiratory disease of the fowl.

uncomplicated and is mainly associated with the degree and duration of action of the primary factor involved. For disease caused by animate primary factors (pathogens) the epidemiology is much more complex and many attributes of the pathogen (e.g. virulence and tropism), and route and weight of infection, as well as intrinsic and extrinsic factors to the fowl are of significance. In certain conditions in which both inanimate factors and pathogens play a part or where more than one pathogen is involved, it may be impossible to classify them into primary and secondary factors.

The transmission of respiratory disease applies only to pathogens and may be direct from host to host or indirect through fomites or other intermediary agents. Direct spread may occur through airborne droplets when birds are in close contact as in intensive management, through the egg from an infected ovary or oviduct and perhaps, but rarely, through infected semen. Transmission is influenced by a number of factors including (1) multiplicity of host species, (2) large numbers of susceptible stock in close contact, (3) the survival of the causal agent within the host and the frequency of its excretion, (4) the survival of the pathogen outside the host, (5) routes of infection, (6) movement of infected stock and fomites. Various management practices such as the siting of houses, ventilation, condition of litter and general hygiene will be of significance in disease spread.

PRIMARY CAUSAL FACTORS

Although such inanimate agents as dietary deficiency (e.g. vitamin A deficiency), excess ammonia, trauma and other factors may be influenced by secondary factors in causing respiratory signs and lesions, their epidemiology is relatively uncomplicated and will not be considered further.

Pathogens, however, because of their varying biological properties and ability to spread have a considerable influence on epidemiology.

Newcastle disease (ND)

Newcastle disease virus is a member of the Paramyxovirus group of the Paramyxoviridae. Its virulence varies among strains from high (velogenic), causing severe disease, to very mild (lentogenic) in which disease may be inapparent. Tropism is also shown by strains of ND viruses (NDV) which may show particular tropism for the respiratory system (pneumotropic), the viscera (visceratropic) or nervous tissue (neurotropic) but all affect the other tissues to some extent. Birds may be carriers of NDV for many months, while the virus can survive outside the body for some weeks unless exposed to disinfectants, high temperatures or direct sunlight. Some resistance in the host is associated with genetic constitution and maturity but more significant protection is associated with the immune response (maternal antibody in the chick and immunity following field infection or vaccination).

Synergy may occur between Newcastle disease virus and influenza A virus and with pathogenic strains of *Escherichia coli* and/or *M. gallisepticum* or *M. synoviae*. "Coli-septicaemia" of broilers may result from infection with *E. coli* and either one or both of the other pathogens. Deficiency of vitamin A and deprivation of food and water for as little as 24 hours, for chicks, exacerbates the resulting respiratory disease caused by NDV. Ammonia in the environment, even in quantities as little as 20 ppm, for four to six weeks adversely influences the effect of NDV on the respiratory system. Exposure to excessive amounts of dust may also result in more severe respiratory disease than with NDV alone.

The ambient temperature can influence the manifestation of ND and under controlled conditions respiratory signs seem to be more frequent at low temperatures, at least for some strains of virus.

Birds in the incubative stage of the disease and those clinically affected are the greatest source of virus. Such virus may be transmitted by movement of the live host or carcases of infected birds. It may be wind-borne or carried on the hands of attendants, and on implements, utensils and clothing. It is important to appreciate that many avian species apart from the fowl are susceptible. Carrier birds of NDV can also be a source of infection.

Infectious bronchitis (IB)

Avian infectious bronchitis virus (IBV) belongs to the Corona-viridae and a number of antigenically different strains are recognized with a variation of virulence. All strains will cause disease of the respiratory system although some appear to be nephrotropic. Following natural infection, IBV has not been recovered from fowl for longer than seven weeks but apparent cycling of infection from bird to bird in a flock may last months. Resistance is influenced by age since severe tracheitis with mortality is only likely to be seen in the very young chick. However, the greatest protection is associated with the immune response.

Among extrinsic influencing factors, concomitant infection with other pathogens is particularly important. A summative or synergistic effect may result from dual infection with IBV and ILT virus. Some strains of avian adenovirus increase the severity and duration of respiratory disease associated with IBV and infection with IBV, adenovirus and *M. gallisepticum* can produce a disease similar in severity and signs to acute ILT. IBV has a synergistic association with *H. paragallinarum*, while with certain strains of *E. coli* alone, or together with *M. gallisepticum* or *M. synoviae*, "coli septicaemia" or a chronic respiratory disease may result.

Excess environmental ammonia (as little as 25–50 ppm) will increase the severity of IBV infection as will a suboptimal brooding temperature for young chickens.

The most usual methods of spread are direct airborne transmission, from fowl to fowl in a flock, and from one flock to another. Fomite transmission may also occur.

Infectious laryngotracheitis (ILT)

This virus belongs to the Herpesviridae. It is of varying virulence; the very mild type causes little or no evidence of disease while the very severe form may cause as much as 50 to 70 per cent mortality in infected stock. The organism affects only the respiratory tract and death results from asphyxia. A proportion of recovered birds become carriers, the organism existing in the trachea for as long as two years. Outside the body the virus can survive for several weeks under farm conditions.

Intrinsic influencing factors include genetic constitution (heavy breeds are more severely affected than light breeds), sex (males are more susceptible than females) and immune status (protection, partial or complete, may follow recovery from infection or vaccination). Of the extrinsic factors the viruses of ILT and IB together have a summation or synergistic effect. Synergism also occurs between ILT and *H. paragallinarum*, and between ILT and *M. gallisepticum*. Deficiency of vitamin A exacerbates the effect of ILT infection while at an ambient temperature of 37°C mortality from ILT is greater than at 20°C.

Spread can occur directly from infected birds either in the incubation or clinical stage of disease or carriers. The virus can also be transmitted on fomites.

Fowl pox

Fowl pox belongs to the genus *Avipox* of the family Poxviridae. Strains vary in virulence and, while tropism has not been shown to occur, in some outbreaks laryngitis with caseous exudate is more common than the classical form of fowl pox with pock lesions on the skin. The virus can survive in scabs, away from the host, for many years.

The only intrinsic factors which appear to exert an influence on the production of disease are age (the young are most susceptible) and the immune status (infection or vaccination results in protection although this may not always be of high degree or long lasting). Of the extrinsic factors, multiple infections involving fowl pox and other pathogens have not received much attention but under field conditions concurrent infection with *H. paragallinarum* causes more severe disease than either pathogen alone.

Because the virus can survive for long periods away from the host, a contaminated environment is a potent source of infection. The organism may gain access through abrasions in the skin as in pecking and mechanically through mosquito bites.

Influenza A infection

The influenza A virus belongs to the Orthomyxoviridae and there are numerous subtypes based on haemagglutinin and neuroaminidase antigens. There is considerable variation in virulence irrespective of subtype. The young chicken is more susceptible than older birds and natural infection or vaccination can give rise to an immune response which may be protective against the same subtype.

Direct spread of virus from bird to bird occurs very rapidly but sources of infection are often undetermined. Migratory birds, especially waterfowl, may be reservoirs of infection.

Avian adenovirus and reovirus infections

Some strains of avian adeno- and reoviruses cause mild respiratory disease under certain experimental conditions. However, they are rarely primary causal agents under field conditions and are more likely to exacerbate other respiratory disease or to show a synergistic effect, for instance, with ND virus, *E. coli* and *M. gallisepticum*.

Pasteurella multocida

At least 16 serotypes of *P. multocida* have been demonstrated by precipitation tests. Isolates vary considerably in virulence irrespective of the strain. Some recovered fowl become carriers but outside the host the organism is very susceptible to drying or to coal tar and other disinfectants. Disease occurs more commonly in adult or nearly adult stock than in younger birds. However, experimental infection by the parenteral route suggests that younger birds are more susceptible. The immune status may be of considerable importance and recovered birds develop protection against further infection by the specific strain.

The combination of *P. multocida* with *H. paragallinarum* is synergistic. Deprivation of food and water for some hours before infection, or exposure to a high temperature (37°C) rather than a low one (20°C) causes chickens to be affected more severely.

Recovered, carrier birds and clinically infected stock and rats may be sources of infection. Airborne infection seems to be unimportant except over very short distances but water troughs may facilitate transmission.

Haemophilus paragallinarum

Antigenic variation occurs among strains of this organism and considerable variation in virulence. A proportion of recovered birds become carriers but the organism survives outside the body for only a few days even in very cold climates. Adult stock are most severely affected and recovered birds are immune for at least several months. Multiple infections with IBV, ILTV, fowl pox, *P. multocida* or *M. gallisepticum* are synergistic and cold, wet conditions predispose to more severe disease. Transmission of infection is mainly associated with carrier birds and those showing clinical signs.

Escherichia coli

Few strains of *E. coli* are probably involved in respiratory disease of fowl and it is invariably in association with other pathogens such as NDV, IBV, *M. gallisepticum* and *M. synoviae*. Such infections may result in "coli-septicaemia".

The organisms are ubiquitous, are found in the upper respiratory tract and intestines of normal birds and can survive for many weeks in dry poultry litter.

Mycoplasma gallisepticum (Mg)

Variation in virulence occurs among isolates, carrier birds exist and the organisms probably survive outside the body for no more than a few days. Very young chicks seem to be most susceptible, especially when infected as embryos, and resistance increases with age. Some degree of protection follows infection or vaccination. *M. gallisepticum* causes most severe respiratory disease when in association with such pathogens as NDV, IBV, ILTV, influenza A, avian adenovirus

and reovirus, *H. paragallinarum* or *E. coli* and often with more
than one of these pathogens concomitantly. Trauma such as
scarification of the trachea, excess ammonia and social stress
such as may occur under intensive management, exacerbate
disease.

Transmission is mainly by direct means such as through
the egg, infected semen or by infected airborne droplets from
carriers or infected birds to others in close contact.

M. synoviae (Ms)

Strains of this organism vary in virulence and also in tropism
for joints and bursae or respiratory tissue. Carriers are found
among recovered stock and survival of the organism away
from the host is probably of short duration under farm
conditions. Recovery from infection may be followed by
increased resistance but multiple infections with NDV or IBV
are synergistic and may, in fact, be necessary to precipitate
clinical disease with *M. synoviae*. Low environmental temperatures increase the incidence and severity of air sacculitis in
three- to four-week old chickens. The spread of infection is
similar to that for *M. gallisepticum*.

Aspergillus fumigatus

Although several species of *Aspergillus* have been associated
with respiratory disease of the fowl, *A. fumigatus* is the most
commonly involved. These fungi are ubiquitous and thrive
in poultry buildings on a variety of poultry food and litter
and in hatcheries. The fungus is toxigenic.

Very young chicks are more susceptible than older birds
and a heavy infection and/or some debility such as with
a dietary deficiency are often of importance in disease
production.

Syngamus trachea

This nematode, in the larval form, is found in the lungs and,
in the adult form, in the trachea and bronchi. The male is

firmly attached to the tracheal wall and is in almost permanent copulation with the female. Large numbers of these parasites cause dyspnoea, coughing and, frequently, asphyxia in young chickens.

Infection may occur directly by the ingestion of either embryonated eggs or larvae by susceptible chicks but most often occurs following the ingestion of infected earthworms or certain molluscs. Only young chickens up to about eight weeks of age are susceptible.

Multiple infections

Many respiratory conditions in the fowl may be associated with more than one causal agent and amelioration or exacerbation may be effected by factors which are intrinsic and/or extrinsic to the chicken.

DIAGNOSIS (Table 3.2)

Features to be considered in diagnosis are clinical signs in the individual and the flock; history of disease in the flock and perhaps neighbouring flocks; lesions (gross and sometimes histological); and demonstration of the causal agent. For pathogens this frequently requires isolation and identification or sometimes an indication of their presence (perhaps in retrospect) by the examination of acute and convalescent sera.

There are few conditions in which respiratory signs and gross lesions of the respiratory tract are alone pathognomonic. However, in a flock with respiratory disease the expectoration of blood, the presence of caseous plugs obstructing the larynx and/or syrinx region or haemorrhagic tracheal casts together with gasping respiration is very strongly suggestive of ILT. Similarly, an acute respiratory disease in which there is marked nasal discharge and swelling of the infraorbital sinuses with frothy conjunctivitis indicates *H. paragallinarum* infection. A tentative diagnosis may be made of *A. fumigatus* infection in brooding chicks which show gasping respiration, no râles and caseous plaque-like lesions with aerial hyphae in the

Table 3.2 Diagnosis of respiratory diseases of the fowl.

Primary causal agent	Respiratory signs and gross lesions of value in differentiating respiratory diseases	Other signs and gross lesions of value in diagnosis	Mortality, prevalence and spread among fowl in a susceptible flock	Confirmation isolation and/or identification of the causal agent	Serological tests
Vitamin A deficiency	Thin dry membrane of necrotic tissue covering the mucous surface of the trachea and bronchi, sometimes sloughed into the lumen	Caseous plaques beneath nicitating membranes; pinhead white lesions on the exits of the mucous glands of the oesophagus; nephritis with visceral gout	Mortality only in advanced cases; sporadic initially but more birds affected with continuing deficiency	Analysis for vitamin A on fresh liver (the lesions resolve on administration of vitamin A)	
Ammonia	None pathognomonic	Conjunctivitis	No mortality; whole flock affected	Smell of ammonia. Estimation of ammonia in the atmosphere	
Newcastle disease virus	None pathognomonic	Diarrhoea, nervous signs especially in young chicks; rapid fall in egg production which does not completely recover; shell-less eggs early in disease	Rapidly spreading from bird to bird and flock to flock, some mortality especially in chicks except in the very mild infections; high mortality in the acute forms of disease	Tracheal and cloacal swabs or macerated trachea and lungs inoculated into the AC of fertile eggs. Identity by HA and HI	HI, SN, ELISA

Agent	Clinical signs	Effect on egg production	Mortality/spread	Laboratory diagnosis	Serology
Infectious bronchitis virus	None pathognomonic	Rapid fall in egg production which does not completely recover; drop in egg quality about one month after infection	Rapidly spreading as in ND	Tracheal swab or macerated trachea and lungs inoculated into the AC of fertile eggs; several passages may be necessary to give death, stunting, or excess renal urates. Scrapings from the trachea may be examined for virus by EM or IF and such examinations can be applied to centrifuged deposits of AF following inoculation and incubation of fertile eggs as above. Identify by SN	HI, SN, ELISA, AGP, IF
Infectious laryngotracheitis virus	Dyspnoea, with cyanosis of the face; high pitched squawk on expiration; coughing up blood; caseous exudate and blood in the trachea and bronchi often in form of casts or plugs	Rapid fall in egg production which returns to normal on recovery of the birds	Mortality varies (0–70%); rapid spread in a susceptible flock: spread from flock to flock capricious	Tracheal swabs inoculated onto the CAM or into the AC of fertile eggs or cell cultures. Identify by IF, EM, AGP or intranuclear inclusions. Alternative examinations include tracheal exudates by AGP or tracheal sections for intranuclear inclusions	SN in fertile eggs or cell culture, ELISA, IF

Table 3.2 Continued.

Primary causal agent	Respiratory signs and gross lesions of value in differentiating respiratory diseases	Other signs and gross lesions of value in diagnosis	Mortality, prevalence and spread among fowl in a susceptible flock	Confirmation isolation and/or identification of the causal agent	Serological tests
Fowl pox virus	Lesions in larynx only	Pocks on comb and face and diphtheritic lesions in oropharynx	Mortality in the laryngeal form usually low and spreads slowly	Similar methods to those for ILT; inclusions are intracytoplasmic	SN in fertile eggs or cell culture
Influenza A virus	None pathognomonic	None, or diarrhoea, nervous signs or fall in egg production	Mortality variable; rapid spread (very high mortality after a short period of illness in the peracute form; no mortality in the very mild form)	Tracheal and cloacal swabs inoculated into the AC of fertile eggs; several passages may be necessary. Identify by HA not neutralized by NDV antiserum and AGP	HI, AGP, ELISA, SN
Pasteurella multicoda "fowl cholera"	None pathognomonic	Swelling of the wattles and leg and wing joints	Mortality variable. Rapid spread from bird to bird in a flock	Tracheal and visceral swabs sown onto blood agar medium and MacConkey. Identify by colony and cell morphology and biochemical tests	

H. paragallinarum "coryza"	Marked nasal discharge, conjunctivitis with frothy exudate, sinusitis	Swelling of the whole face	No mortality in uncomplicated cases; very rapid spread	Examine stained smears of exudate. Tracheal and infraorbital sinus swabs sown onto media containing NAD (can be provided by *Staphyloccus* feeder culutre), increased carbon dioxide atmosphere. Identify by colony and cell morphology and biochemical tests	RSA, TA
E. coli (respiratory disease mainly associated with multiple infection)	Caseous thickening of the air sac walls	Caseous pericarditis; fibrinous peri-hepatitis in intensively housed young growers	Of sporadic occurrences in a flock	Swabs from lesions sown onto agar. Identify by colony and cell morphology and biochemical tests; pathogenicity studies involve i/v inoculation of 4 w.o. chicks	None
M. gallisepticum and *M. synoviae*	None pathognomonic. Respiratory disease mainly associated with multiple infections	Caseous air sacculitis in some forms	Little mortality from the respiratory disease in natural uncomplicated infections. Infection in very young chicks usually rapidly spreading within a flock; variable speed of spread in older birds	Swabs from nares, infraorbital sinus, trachea or air sac onto/into mycoplasma media. Identification by colony morphology followed by IF or GI DNA probes	RSA, HI, IF

Table 5.2 Avian anthelmintics.

Active ingredient	Trade name/source	Administration	Indications
Levamisole	Nilverm; Pitman-Moore	In drinking water or by injection	Gut roundworms
Piperazine	Spartakon; Harkers Janssen	Tablets	Gut roundworms in pigeons
	Citrazine; Loveridge	In drinking water	Gut roundworms especially ascarids
Thiabendazole	Thibenzole; MSD AGVET	Powder or premix in feed	Syngamus species in pheasants
Mebendazole	Mebenvet; Janssen	In feed	Gut roundworms, Syngamus species and tapeworms (not recommended for pigeons or parrots)
Cambendazole	Ascapilla; Univet	Capsules	Gut roundworms in pigeons

trachea, lung and air sacs. *S. trachea* infection can be confirmed simply by demonstrating the nematodes in the trachea.

When the respiratory and other signs and lesions are taken together with mortality, prevalence and transmission of disease then many conditions may be differentiated when they appear in typical form. They include vitamin A deficiency, ND in very young chicks showing nervous signs or ataxia, loss of control of the head and neck and walking backwards, ILT except in the very mild form, fowl cholera in which some birds show swelling of the wattles (Fig. 3.6), and *E. coli* infection which in multiple infection with NDV, IB, Mg or Ms cause "coli-septicaemia", with the pathognomonic lesions of the pericardium, air sacs and liver. However, the varying disease picture resulting from variation in virulence and tropism of pathogens, differing immune status of birds and flocks and other influencing factors including multiple infections, make confirmation of diagnosis necessary. Some of the more commonly recommended techniques used in confirmation are listed although they are by no means comprehensive.

CONTROL (Table 3.3)

The general principles of disease control comprise: (1) prevention or limitation of contact between the host and the causal

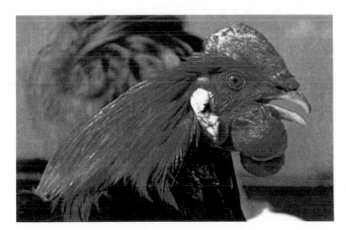

Fig. 3.6
Chronically swollen wattles resulting from *P. multocida* infection.

Table 3.3 Control of respiratory diseases of fowl.

Primary causal agent	Some specific control measures
Vitamin A deficiency	Administration of vitamin A in food
Ammonia	Provide conditions conducive to dry litter and adequate ventilation
Newcastle disease virus	(a) Immunization: attenuated live virus vaccine at three weeks—also at day-old if risk is high Less attenuated live virus vaccine at 6, 10 and 18 weeks or inactivated vaccine at 18 weeks (b) Eradication: Flocks, from which virus has been isolated and/or reactor birds have been found serologically, are slaughtered
Infectious bronchitis virus	Immunization: attenuated live virus vaccine at 3 and 8 weeks. Less attenuated live virus vaccine or inactivated virus vaccine at 18 weeks
Infectious laryngotracheitis virus	Immunization: attenuated strain by eye drop between 16 and 18 weeks. Also at 3 weeks if risk is high
Fowl pox virus	Immunization: (a) Mild disease: mild strain such as pigeon pox virus given by scarification between 6 and 18 weeks (b) Severe disease: fowl pox virus given by wing-web stab between 6 and 18 weeks
Influenza A virus	(a) Immunization: antigenic diversity among subtypes and strains within subtypes limits value of vaccination. However, inactivated autogenous virus grown in chick embryos may reduce losses (b) Eradication of highly pathogenic avian influenza viruses: Many countries legislate against introduction and spread of these viruses which includes slaughter and disposal of affected and in contact poultry (c) Housing and management, to prevent the introduction of infection (especially from wild birds) and to prevent spread, is advocated

P. multocida	(a)	Spread from potential reservoirs of infection, as sick birds, carriers, rats and wild birds, should be prevented as far as possible
	(b)	Drug therapy: variety of drugs and antibiotics are effective but drug sensitivity should be determined. Following cessation of treatment resurgence of disease may occur
	(c)	Immunization: inactivated vaccines used with some success; autogenous vaccines are more protective
H. paragallinarum	(a)	Introduction of carrier birds should be prevented
	(b)	Immunization: bacterins prepared from killed whole cultures given intramuscularly, on two occasions, at three weeks apart between 10 and 19 weeks of age, provide some protection
	(c)	Drug therapy: variety of drugs and antibiotics are effective but drug sensitivity should be determined. Following cessation of treatment relapses occur
E. coli	(a)	Control intercurrent pathogens (e.g. IBV and mycoplasmas)
	(b)	Drug therapy for *E. coli* including furan and sulpha drugs, ampicillin, quinolones and many other antibiotics; drug sensitivity should be determined
M. gallisepticum and *M. synoviae*	(a)	Drug therapy: for treatment of hatching eggs and birds; tylosin, gentamicin, tiamulin, lincomycin, spectinomycin, spiromycin, quinolones and other antibiotics have been found of value
	(b)	Eradication: hatching eggs are treated with antibiotics or "heat treated" and flocks regularly monitored. Flocks in which reactors are found are not used for breeding
	(c)	Immunization: attenuated live strains have been used for *M. gallisepticum* vaccination of young chickens
A. fumigatus		Mouldy litter and mould contaminated food or implements should be avoided
S. trachea		Chickens should be prevented access to infected hosts especially the earthworm
		Drug therapy: tetramisole hydrochloride and thibendazole

agent; (2) increasing resistance of host to the pathogen; (3) treatment of host to minimize adverse effects of the pathogen on the host and to limit transmission; and (4) avoiding or reducing the effect of predisposing factors.

For the control of conditions caused by inanimate agents the application of the principles (apart from (2) and (3) above) is relatively uncomplicated. However, for disease caused by living organisms control is more involved and usually requires an application of several of them concomitantly.

MINIMIZING CONTACT OF HOST AND CAUSAL AGENT

Minimizing contact between the fowl and the pathogen should be practised by all means within the scope of profitable poultry production and, when feasible, eradication of the pathogen may be attempted. Some practical considerations in preventing or limiting contact between the host and the pathogen are given.

General

Buildings

Buildings should be sited in relative isolation (100 m from other poultry stock and highways) especially those with wire-mesh sides. They should be constructed so as to be readily cleaned and disinfected and inaccessible to wild birds and vermin. Buildings, together with equipment and utensils, should be cleaned, disinfected and "rested" between successive groups of birds. Positive pressure, filtered air ventilation (air entering through a glass fibre ceiling) may be of value in reducing infection for "controlled environment houses".

"All in/all out" management

An "all in/all out" policy for the whole premises should be followed if practicable but certainly for individual houses and for broiler production.

Species, ages and sources of stock

Different avian species, age groups and birds from different sources should not be housed together, and once established a flock should be "closed" for its productive life.

Litter

Fresh litter should be provided for each new group of birds.

Food and water

Food and water should be provided from such sources and by such means that there is no opportunity for contamination with avian pathogens.

Personnel

Personnel should wear protective clothing and boots, and facilities should be available for washing hands and cleaning boots between different groups of fowls. Personnel should take practicable precautions to minimize the carriage of infective material on hands, boots and clothing, etc.

Hatching eggs and hatcheries

The management of hatching eggs and hatcheries is probably of greatest importance with reference to respiratory pathogens like *E. coli* and *A. fumigatus* which might gain access to the embryo through the shell or to the chick on hatching.

Eggs

Only clean eggs should be used for hatching and should be collected frequently (five times per day). Eggs should be fumigated with formaldehyde gas as soon as possible after collection and stored under clean conditions. Nest boxes should also be kept in a clean condition.

Hatchery

The hatchery design and management should allow only one way movement of air and eggs (from reception to setter to hatcher to despatch of chicks and disposal of waste). The premises should be clean, disinfected regularly and monitored frequently for infection. The hatcher and hatcher room should be cleaned and disinfected immediately after a hatch and before reception of the next group of eggs. The hatch debris should be removed from the premises with care.

Newly hatched chicks

Chicks should be examined and sexed in as clean an environment as possible, and despatched in clean boxes in a disinfected vehicle.

Eradication policy

For the control of some avian respiratory pathogens, an eradication policy has been found practicable. In the practice of such a policy, minimizing contact between the host and causal organism is essential and, apart from the methods already discussed, the importance of stock movement restrictions must be emphasized. This may apply to a country, a district or to a premises, and importation restrictions and movement restrictions may be imposed on live fowl, carcases or products. It may be necessary also to slaughter and adequately dispose of infected and in-contact stock, and to clean and disinfect premises afterwards.

Monitoring for freedom from infection should be undertaken periodically, usually serologically, but sometimes by attempted isolation and identification of the causal organism (e.g. mycoplasmas).

In considering an eradication policy as part of a country's legislation it is important to appreciate the significance of diagnostic methods adequate to recognize infection before it is widely disseminated.

For conditions which are not highly contagious (e.g. mycoplasmosis), breeders have imposed eradication policies on their own flocks. For highly invasive conditions, like Newcastle disease, however, national legislation is necessary and is practised in several countries.

INCREASING RESISTANCE OF HOST TO PATHOGEN

Increasing the resistance of the host to the pathogen implies vaccination, using live or inactivated vaccines or both. Inactivated vaccines are given parenterally but live vaccines may be given by a number of routes including coarse spray for day-old chicks, beak dipping, drinking water, eye drop, aerosol, scarification of the skin (fowl pox), scarification of the cloaca (ILT) or wing stab (mesogenic Newcastle disease and fowl pox vaccines).

Any flock to be vaccinated should be in good health. The vaccine should be potent, safe and uncontaminated and administered so that its potency is not neutralized by disinfectants or adverse environmental factors. Furthermore, the method of administration should be appropriate to the age, immune status, numbers and management of the fowl. If there is the likelihood of the vaccine precipitating a respiratory complex disease like "coli septicaemia", drug therapy may be practised to preclude the worst effects. Immuno-suppressive infections may adversely affect the protection obtained from vaccination and perhaps increase the susceptibility of the stock to live vaccines.

TREATMENT

Treatment consists of the use of drugs and antibiotics, either prophylactically or therapeutically, in those conditions associated with bacteria or mycoplasmas. This includes drugs used for "egg-dipping" or egg inoculation in mycoplasma infections. For fowls, mass administration is usually practised when drugs are included in the food or drinking water.

AVOIDING PREDISPOSING FACTORS

This may involve precautions against any of the extrinsic influencing factors listed above. The general measures described above are applied as appropriate to the control of the various respiratory diseases of the fowl but the more common specific methods relative to the primary causal agents are outlined above.

FURTHER READING

Anon. (1980) *Isolation and Identification of Avian Pathogens*, 2nd edn, (eds Hitchener, S. B. and others). New York, American Association of Avian Pathologists. Creative Printing Company Inc.

Anon. (1981) *Avian Immunology, Proceedings of the 16th Poultry Science Symposium 25–27 September 1980* (eds Rose, M. E. and others). Edinburgh, British Poultry Science Ltd.

Calnek, B. W., Barnes, H. J., Beard, C. W., Reid, W. M. and Yoder, H. W. (1991) (eds) *Diseases of Poultry*, 9th edn. London, Wolfe Publications.

Gross, W. B. and Colmano, G. (1971) *Poultry Science* **100**, 1213.

Jordan, F. T. W. (1972) *Veterinary Record* **90**, 556.

Jordan, F. T. W. (1990) (ed.) *Poultry Diseases*, 3rd edn. London, Baillière Tindall.

CHAPTER 4

Parasitic Conditions in Poultry 1: Protozoal Diseases

A. J. TREES

This chapter concentrates on protozoal diseases of poultry, their diagnosis and control. Chapter 5 will go on to deal with helminths and arthropods.

INTRODUCTION

Coccidiosis is an important disease of poultry caused primarily by protozoa of the genus *Eimeria*. Infection with most *Eimeria* species is confined to the gut, although renal coccidiosis associated with *E. truncata* can be a severe disease in young geese. *Eimeria* species are highly host specific but within each host there may be several different pathogenic species. Coccidiosis is of greatest importance in intensive rearing systems where high stocking densities predispose to the accumulation of high environmental populations of the causal organism.

COCCIDIOSIS IN CHICKENS

Worldwide, coccidiosis is one of the three or four most important diseases in chickens. Its economic impact is difficult to quantify accurately but, in the UK, current annual expenditure on prophylactic drugs alone, amounts to approximately £5.25 million.

The major species which infect chickens along with their characteristics are shown in Table 4.1. Oocysts passed in faeces become infective after sporulation in a minimum period of 12 to 18 hours under warm, moist and well aerated conditions. Infection is followed by a period of massive multiplication in epithelial and subepithelial cells which culminates in the shedding of oocysts in faeces from four to five days after infection. Within a short time in susceptible stock heavy environmental contamination can result.

The degree of pathology and disease is.dependent on both the species of *Eimeria* involved and the size of the infecting dose of oocysts. Infection, especially at continuous low levels— so called "trickle infection"—induces a strong degree of protective immunity which is specific for each *Eimeria* species. Day-old chicks do not appear to derive any passively transferred protective immunity from the hen via the egg.

In a growing flock of susceptible birds there is an unseen race between the acquisition of flock immunity by low grade

Table 4.1 *Eimeria* species of chickens.

Species	Pathogenicity	Main site of lesions	Type of lesion
E. tenella	High	Caecum	Haemorrhagic, caecal core
E. necatrix	High	Mid-intestine	Focal haemorrhagic and pale lesions; ballooning
E. brunetti	High	Posterior intestine	Haemorrhage
E. maxima	Medium/high	Mid-intestine	Focal, haemorrhagic
E. acervulina	Medium	Duodenum	Pale, striated
E. praecox	Low	Duodenum	Inapparent
E. mitis	Low	Mid-intestine	Inapparent

NB There is evidence that *E. mivati*, which is referred to in most textbooks, is not a valid species.

infection and the build-up of the parasite population. Should factors favour the parasite, such as an initial high degree of contamination and good conditions for oocyst sporulation (e.g. wet litter) then clinical disease may occur most typically at 3–6 weeks old.

More often, flock immunity will be acquired without clinical signs though there may be economically important impairment of growth and feed conversion. Outbreaks of disease can occur at over 6 weeks old especially with certain species of *Eimeria* or in any situation where waning flock immunity coincides with challenge, e.g. if floor-reared birds are caged for a period, thus preventing reinfection and the boosting of immunity, then suddenly re-exposed to infection. Alternatively, certain anticoccidials will prevent the acquisition of immunity so that when drugs are withdrawn, birds are susceptible to challenge.

DIAGNOSIS

Eimeria species show a remarkable degree of tropism for certain parts of the alimentary tract and also vary in the nature of the lesions produced (Fig. 4.1). Thus, species responsible for an outbreak of disease can usually be identified without difficulty. However, mixed infections commonly occur presenting a more complicated post mortem picture. Disease is characterized by diarrhoea with, in some cases, dysentery. Bloody droppings with an increase in mortality will be the signs of a severe outbreak caused by *E. tenella*, *E. brunetti*, or *E. necatrix*. *E. maxima* can also cause clinical illness with characteristic salmon pink droppings. Other species may cause mild clinical signs, diarrhoea or a check in growth.

Diagnosis is confirmed by post mortem examination. Characteristic lesions will usually be noticeable from the serosal surface but the intestine should be opened and the mucosa carefully examined. The presence of parasites in mucosal scrapings in association with typical lesions is diagnostic (Fig. 4.2). Parasites are easily identified in unstained wet smears either as oocysts or clumps of schizonts with free merozoites. If birds are examined during the acute phase of disease oocysts may not be found but schizonts and merozoites are abundant. It is worth noting that heavy infections may

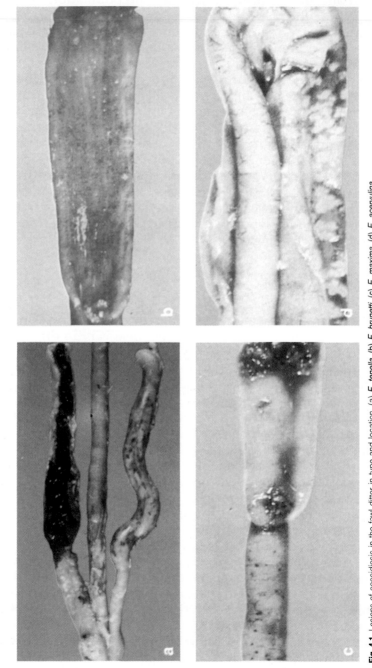

Fig. 4.1 Lesions of coccidiosis in the fowl differ in type and location. (a) *E. tenella*, (b) *E. brunetti*, (c) *E. maxima*, (d) *E. acervulina*.

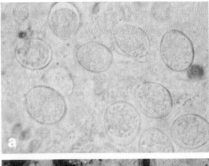
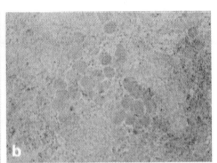
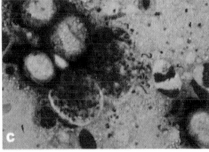

Fig. 4.2
Diagnosis of coccidiosis in the fowl is confirmed by the detection of parasites in mucosal scrapings. (a) Oocysts, (b) clumps of schizonts (low power). In Giemsa-stained smears (c), mature gametocytes show dark stained granules. Smaller oocysts do not take the stain.

occur concurrently with other disease conditions (such as salmonellosis, infectious bursitis or clostridial disease) as a secondary, rather than a primary pathogen. It is important for accurate diagnosis that fresh carcases are examined as lesions may become obscure post mortem.

Finally, because the majority of young flocks will be receiving anticoccidial medication, an investigation of an outbreak should include the assay of feed for anticoccidial drugs. Feed samples representative of the feed offered five to 10 days before clinical disease should be examined. Many outbreaks are a result of suboptimal inclusion of drug or failure to include it all. If recommended levels of drug are shown to have been available then drug resistance should be considered.

CONTROL

It is impossible under commercial conditions to prevent infection completely. Sporulated oocysts are resistant to commonly used disinfectants (they are susceptible only to small molecular weight and highly toxic agents like ammonia or methyl bromide) and survive many months under normal conditions of temperature and humidity. With good hygiene it is possible to rear broilers without medication or by using a cheap anticoccidial of modest efficacy and not suffer clinical disease. This will be an economic decision not without risk!

In most cases it will be advisable to rear broilers with anticoccidial prophylactic drugs in the feed. Apart from preventing clinical disease this may prove economically beneficial due to the effective control of subclinical infection.

A summary of currently used drugs in the UK is shown in Table 4.2 (for a summary of anticoccidials for all host species, see Gregory and Norton (1986) *In Practice* **8**, p. 33). The most widely used drugs are all ionophorous antibiotics. These have proved highly efficacious. They are, however, potentially toxic to both target and non-target animals. Moreover, there are toxic interactions between some ionophores and certain antibiotics, and it is important that farmers, as well as veterinarians, are aware of these.

Drug resistance is a problem that has reduced the effectiveness of many older, and some new, anticoccidials. Resistance among chicken coccidia to the ionophores has been very slow to develop, although there is now evidence that resistance is occurring in some locations.

Outbreaks of disease may be treated with sulphonamides, furaltadone or amprolium. Rapid intervention is essential, so water medication is usually preferred. The economic costs of an outbreak will be substantial even if therapy is effective and the need to resort to medication indicates a need to review prophylactic measures.

There is no vaccine for coccidiosis currently available in the UK. Uncontrolled immunoprophylaxis is practised for layer and breeder replacements by rearing under decreasing "step-down" doses of anticoccidial or with drugs of modest efficacy which permit the acquisition of immunity by natural infection. In these cases drugs can be completely withdrawn well before point of lay.

There is increasing research interest in a vaccine and two aproaches utilizing live oocysts are under development. The first, developed by researchers at the Houghton Laboratory, IADR, uses oocysts attenuated by repeated selection of the earliest oocysts shed after infection to produce so called

Table 4.2 Anticoccidials for prevention of disease in chickens by administration in feed.

Type of compound	Generic name	Trade name	Source	Dose (ppm)	Withdrawal period (days)
Polyether ionophorous antibiotics	Monensin	Elancoban and others	Elanco and others	100–120	3
	Narasin	Monteban	Elanco	70	5
	Lasalocid	Avatec	Hoffman la Roche	75–125	5
	Salinomycin	Sacox	Hoechst	60	5
Amprolium combinations	Amprolium + ethopobate	Amprolmix	MSD	125+8	3
	Amprolium + ethopabate + sulpha-quinoxaline	Pancoxin	MSD	varies	7
Nitrobenzamides	Dinitolmide	Various	Various	62.5–125	3
Sulphonamides	Sulpha-quinoxaline	Embasin Premix	May & Baker	125	5
Pyridones	Clopidol	Coyden and others	Dow and others	125	5
	Clopidol + methyl benzcquate	Lerbek	Dow	100 + 8.35	5
Quinolones	Decoquinate	Deccox	May & Baker	20–40	3
Guanidines	Robenidine	Cycostat	Cyanamid	33	5
	Nicarbazin	Nicrazin	MSD	125	7
	Halofuginone	Stenorol	Hoechst	3	5

"precocious strains". Strains of all seven significant species are included. Another approach under development is to stimulate "trickle" infection by controlled low dose administration of oocysts in feed using a special delivery system.

There is also an increasing amount of research into devising a non-living genetically engineered vaccine but this is a longer term prospect.

COCCIDIOSIS IN TURKEYS (Table 4.3)

Many of the general remarks made about chicken coccidiosis apply to turkey coccidiosis. This is primarily a disease of young poults. Watery diarrhoea is more usual than dysentery. As with coccidiosis in other hosts, diagnosis should not be based solely on post mortem lesion appearance; it is important that parasites be demonstrated in association with the appropriate lesions. Because they occupy the same site, *E. adenoides* and *E. meleagridis* may require careful differentiation. The latter does not cause disease but may produce visible, though non-haemorrhagic, lesions, caecal cores and large numbers of oocysts. The oocysts of the two species are of similar length but those of *E. meleagridis* are wider and have a lower length:width ratio (1.34 compared with 1.54 of *E. adenoides*).

Fewer drugs are registered for anticoccidial use in turkeys than in chickens. It is important to note that some ionophores

Table 4.3 *Eimeria* species of turkeys.

Species	Pathogenicity	Main site of lesions	Type of lesions
E. adenoides	High	Caecum	Petechial haemorrhages Caseous caecal core
E. meleagridis	Low	Caecum	Caseous core
E. meleagrimitis	High	Anterior and mid-intestine	Necrotic enteritis; petechial haemorrhages

are toxic to turkeys even at dose levels recommended for chickens.

Geese

In addition to enteric infections with a variety of species (notably *E. anseris* and *E. nocens*) which can cause disease, geese may also suffer from renal coccidiosis caused by *E. truncata*. This parasite produces severe disease in goslings typified by depression, emaciation, diarrhoea and perhaps death within a few days of the onset of signs. Parasites cause macroscopic lesions in the kidneys and are found in epithelial cells of the kidney tubules.

Ducks

Several *Eimeria* species parasitize ducks. In addition, severe enteric disease in ducklings may be associated with *Tyzzeria perniciosa*. This is readily distinguished from *Eimeria* species since the sporulated oocysts contain eight naked sporozoites rather than four sporocysts of *Eimeria* species.

Gamebirds

In pheasants both intestinal and caecal infections occur, usually resulting from *E. duodenalis*, *E. phasiani* or *E. colchici*. The last named is the most pathogenic causing an enteritis and, in the caeca where the oocysts are produced, caecal cores may form.

Control of coccidiosis in species other than chickens and turkeys is largely dependent on attention to hygiene and on treatment with sulphonamides. Chemoprophylaxis should be attempted only if the drugs are known to be safe for the target species. In game birds, clopidol at 125 ppm in feed has been widely used for chemoprophylaxis. The elimination of damp areas in pens is an important preventive measure.

Sulphonamides are coccidiostatic, so treatment must be maintained for some time preferably in an on/off strategy to allow immunity to develop.

HISTOMONIASIS

Histomoniasis, infectious enterohepatitis or blackhead, as it is variously called, is caused by *Histomonas meleagridis*, a protozoan which infects a variety of gallinaceous birds but is primarily a cause of disease in turkey poults and occasionally game birds and broilers. The parasite invades the caecal mucosa and from there spreads to the liver (Fig. 4.3). In young turkeys the first clinical signs are depression, anorexia and the passing of characteristic sulphur-yellow coloured faeces. A cyanotic head is neither invariable nor unique to this disease so "blackhead" is something of a misnomer. Mortality may be substantial reaching a peak, if untreated, about a week after the onset of clinical signs.

At post mortem examination gross lesions are present in both caecum and liver. In the caecum, a mucosal inflammatory response coinciding with the onset of clinical signs leads to the formation of a caseous caecal core. Liver lesions become grossly apparent within two to three days of the first clinical signs and progressively enlarge. The depressed, circumscribed lesions, comprising an inner necrotic focus surrounded by a parasite-infiltrated, inflammatory zone are pathognomonic. They remain conspicuous long after death. If confirmation of

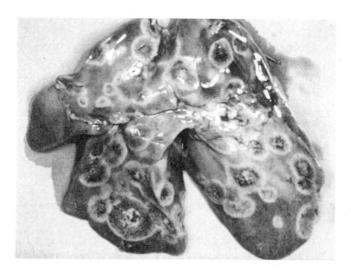

Fig. 4.3
Histomoniasis in a turkey poult. This infection causes characteristic lesions in the liver.

diagnosis is needed, parasites are visible in stained sections from the margins of lesions as rounded up protozoa sur rounded by a vacuole.

Chickens only occasionally show signs of disease but have been historically important as reservoirs of infection for turkeys. The most important route of transmission for *Histomonas*, which itself is a rather delicate organism, is within the eggs of the caecal nematode *Heterakis gallinarum*. Apart from guaranteeing safe passage through the gizzard of the infected host, this collaboration between parasites means that infection can persist for substantial periods in soil. The earthworm may also intervene as a transport host by swallowing the nematode eggs and further enhancing their spread.

Although this disease has become less prevalent with the advent of intensive indoor turkey rearing away from chickens, in-feed chemoprophylaxis may be thought judicious. Dimetridazole may be added to turkey feed for the first few weeks of life. This drug is also available in water soluble form for treatment and can be used in chickens, game birds and guinea fowl as well as turkeys. In free range situations anthelmintic medication against *Heterakis* species may usefully supplement specific antihistomonal treatment.

CRYPTOSPORIDIUM

This parasite is attracting considerable interest as a pathogen of man and animals. In poultry, enteric infections have been encountered from a few days of age, but have been only rarely reported in association with clinical illness. In contrast, there are a number of reports, mainly from the USA, of cryptosporidial infection of the upper respiratory tract associated with morbidity and mortality in a variety of species, including chickens, turkeys, quail and peafowl. Clinical signs have included coughing, dyspnoea and naso-ocular discharges. In Britain, conjunctivitis has been reported due to cryptosporidial infection in pheasants. These clinical cases have occurred in birds of a variety of ages from two to 11 weeks or older. Diagnosis of respiratory tract infection is based on the detection in sections of cryptosporidial organisms (2 to 6 μm diameter) on the surface of the relevant mucosal epithelium. No specific chemotherapy is available.

OTHER PROTOZOA

Although a variety of flagellated protozoa are common commensals of the gut, some are occasionally associated with disease. The causal organisms are probably most easily detected when they are alive and motile in wet smears of intestinal contents. For this to be successful absolutely fresh carcases must be examined. As well as examining wet smears, air-dried smears should be made simultaneously, fixed and stained with Giesma. To avoid the organisms being obscured by debris it may be advisable to dilute the intestinal contents and using serum for this purpose may help reduce distortion in drying. It is best to avoid the tendency to make smears too thick—morphological detail is best seen in thin, rapidly dried smears.

Hexamitiasis, caused by *Hexamita meleagridis* has occasionally been diagnosed as causing enteritis in turkey poults in the UK. The disease has also been reported in pheasants and may be commoner than is thought. At post mortem examination the intestine, especially the upper small intestine, is distended with watery contents. These contain motile *Hexamita* species with six anterior and two posterior flagella. In stained smears, two nuclei can be seen. *Hexamita* species form cysts so, where practicable, environmental hygiene can play a part in prevention. Furazolidone and tetracyclines have been used as medication.

Trichomonads are common commensals of the large intestine and are probably non-pathogenic in chickens but caecal trichomoniasis can be a serious disease in young game birds. Clinical signs include depression, foamy yellow droppings and mortality. On post mortem examination the distended caeca filled with foamy light coloured fluid are characteristic. The causal organisms carry four anterior flagella and a single recurrent posteriorly directed flagellum with an associated undulating membrane. Trichomonads do not form cysts and are transmitted via contaminated feeders and waterers. High stocking densities in moist conditions will predispose to outbreaks. It is possible that infection may be introduced by wild birds to outdoor reared gamebirds. In pheasants, dimetridazole at 60 kg/45 litres drinking water for five days, followed by a further five days treatment at half this dosage has been found effective.

ACKNOWLEDGEMENTS

Dr F. T. W. Jordan is thanked for helpful comments.

CHAPTER 5

Parasitic Conditions in Poultry 2: Helminths and Arthropods

ALEXANDER TREES AND WILLIAM BEESLEY

Chapter 4 concentrated on protozoal diseases of poultry. In this chapter the authors deal with helminths and external parasites.

INTRODUCTION

There is a great variety of helminths infecting poultry in the widest sense of the word and this account is, of necessity, selective. Reference to the detailed host/parasite lists of Soulsby (1982) and Schofield (1983) will be useful in investigating parasitism in less commonly encountered host species.

NEMATODES OF THE RESPIRATORY TRACT

The major pathogenic worm is *Syngamus trachea* which causes the condition of "gapes" in gallinaceous birds (Fig. 5.1). The related species *Cyathostoma bronchialis* causes a similar condition in geese.

S. *trachea* inhabits the trachea of a variety of birds, both wild and domestic. It has been called the Don Juan of

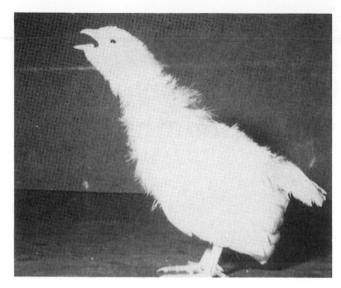

Fig. 5.1
A chick with "gapes",
clinical infection with
Syngamus trachea.

nematodes from its characteristic of dwelling attached to the respiratory mucosa in copulating pairs, the much smaller male giving the whole pair a Y-shaped appearance. Disease is caused by the physical blockage of the respiratory tract; the progressive asphyxiation causes depression, with resting spells interspersed with the characteristic gaping attitude. It is frequently fatal.

The nematode life cycle can be direct or, more importantly, may involve the earthworm. In the earthworm, infections can persist for many years and over a period of time soil can become heavily infected. Moreover, wild birds provide reservoirs of infection for domestic stock.

The disease is seen most often nowadays in game birds and ornamental or zoo birds which are confined to outdoor pens. It has disappeared from chickens and turkeys reared on impervious floors—but like a number of other nematode conditions this is one which can be expected to reappear on farms returning to free-range management systems.

Diagnosis is based on the characteristic clinical signs, history of exposure to sources of infection and the detection of eggs in faeces. Ovoid, with an indistinct polar cap at each end, they are unlike any other egg likely to be encountered except *Capillaria* species which are more rectangular, thicker shelled and with more pronounced polar caps.

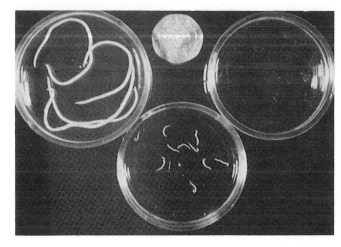

Fig. 5.2
The three main
groups of gut
helminths in poultry
differ greatly in size
and appearance. Left
to right: *Ascaridia*
species, *Heterakis*
species and
Capillaria species.

INTESTINAL NEMATODES

There are three main taxonomic groups of intestinal nematodes of significance—*Capillaria* species, *Heterakis* species and *Ascaridia* species (Fig. 5.2).

Several *Capillaria* species will infect different parts of the intestine of chickens, turkeys and other birds (Table 5.1). Some depend on the earthworm as intermediate host and consequently are restricted to free-range birds. Others have a direct life cycle. *Capillaria* species, although the smallest and least obvious of the intestinal nematodes, are potentially the most pathogenic and can cause severe disease. They must be looked for carefully in mucosal washings under a dissecting microscope at post mortem examination.

Table 5.1 *Capillaria* species of domestic birds in the UK.

Species	Main site	Intermediate host	Comments
Capillaria bursata	Small intestine	Earthworm	Chicken
Capillaria caudinflata	Small intestine	Earthworm	Quite common, various hosts
Capillaria obsignata	Small intestine	None	Common. Various hosts
Capillaria anatis	Caecum	?	Mainly ducks

Heterakis gallinarum is a sturdy white ascarid and is commonplace in the caeca of chickens, turkeys and many other birds. It is probably never a primary cause of clinical disease but is significant because of its role in the epidemiology of histomoniasis. By contrast, the related *H. isolonche*, of pheasants and other game birds, invades the mucosa provoking a nodular typhlitis or enteritis with severe disease and even death (Fig. 5.3). The nodules are grossly visible in the mucosa and harbour worms of various stages including egg-laying adults.

By far the largest nematodes of birds and quite unmistakable, are the *Ascaridia* species which infest the small intestine. *A. galli* of chickens and other birds may be a cause of ill-thrift, enteritis or intestinal impaction in young birds, though as with other ascarids the size of these worms may lead to a false impression of their pathogenicity. The life cycle is direct. Thick shelled typical ascarid eggs are shed in the faeces and may remain infective for months in moist conditions so that debilitating infections can develop in birds on poorly managed deep litter.

OTHER INTESTINAL NEMATODES

Tetrameres fissispina is not of great importance, but it might be encountered at post mortem examination in ducks (Fig.

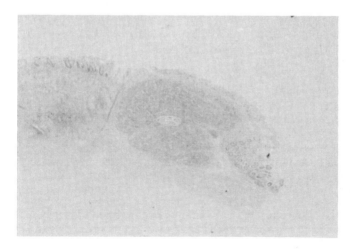

Fig. 5.3
Heterakis isolonche in the pheasant. Unlike *H. gallinarum* in the fowl, this species provokes nodule formation in the gut mucosa.

5.4). The adult females inhabit the glands of the proventriculus and engorge on blood. They can be seen at post mortem examination as dark spots in the mucosa and can be expressed from the glands. They resemble no other nematode, the female being almost spherical. Infections can cause emaciation and anaemia. The life cycle is indirect.

In the gizzard, *Amidostomum anseris* is a parasite quite specific to geese. It can be severely pathogenic in goslings with anorexia, emaciation, anaemia and high mortality. The location of the worm in this host facilitates identification. The life cycle is direct.

In the caecum, in addition to *Heterakis* species, infestations with the much smaller *Trichostrongylus tenuis* may be encountered in a variety of wild and domestic birds. This has a direct life cycle with infection by the ingestion of infective larvae from the environment. It is particularly noteworthy as a pathogen of grouse where it can be responsible for considerable mortality in young birds. Caeca become swollen and inflamed and the small worms (females up to 1 cm long) will be seen by examination of mucosal scrapings.

CESTODES

A vast number of tapeworms have been described from birds and, as far as is known, all require an intermediate host. Never of great pathogenicity, these parasites have become

(a)   (b)

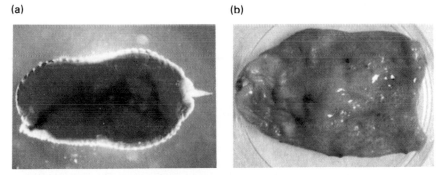

Fig. 5.4 (a) Dark red spots and shadows in the proventricular mucosa in ducks indicate infection with *Tetrameres fissispina*. (b) The adult females, engorged with blood, can be squeezed from the mucosa.

rare in conditions of modern poultry rearing. Should they be encountered and control considered necessary, identification of the worm will indicate the intermediate host involved. Control measures are best directed against this and minor management changes can break the life cycle. Readers are directed to a comprehensive chapter by Reid in Hofstad (1984) for further details.

CONTROL OF HELMINTHIASES

Management practices largely determine the extent and types of helminthiases. Confinement rearing will usually exclude those parasites requiring an intermediate host. The modern practices of rearing single species without mixed age groups has done much to reduce the prevalence of even directly transmitted helminths. On the other hand the increase in pen rearing of game birds, the growth of ornamental or zoological collections and a limited tendency to return to free range systems means that helminthiases are still not uncommonly encountered in these situations. Anthelmintics currently available for use in poultry are listed in Table 5.2. It is important to note that the efficacy and safety of compounds may not have been assessed in minor host species or for parasites of minor economic importance so caution is recommended in such cases.

EXTERNAL PARASITES OF POULTRY

External parasites are often surprisingly hard to find and their real numbers on the host may greatly exceed those seen at first inspection. Poultry in Britain can harbour several genera of lice, three of mites and one species of flea. The problem of external parasites on poultry has completely changed with intensification of the industry. Chicken lice, for example, seldom infest modern layer or broiler units because there is hardly time for large populations of these parasites to build up and any lice which leave the host soon die. Poultry mites, on the other hand, are much more resilient, surviving for

Table 3.2 Continued.

Primary causal agent	Respiratory signs and gross lesions of value in differentiating respiratory diseases	Other signs and gross lesions of value in diagnosis	Mortality, prevalence and spread among fowl in a susceptible flock	Confirmation isolation and/or identification of the causal agent	Serological tests
A. fumigatus "brooder pneumonia"	Gasping respiration without rales; plaque-like caseous lesions with dark brown/green centres of aerial hyphae. Mainly a disease of brooding chickens	Lesions occasionally present in other organs and tissues (e.g. liver, brain, etc.)	Rapid spreading; mortality varies, usually 10–50% of flock of brooding chickens	Examine smear of lesions treated with sodium or potassium hydroxide. Swab of lesion sown onto Sabouraud's medium. Identify fungus	None
S. trachea "gapes"	Characteristic round worms in the trachea	None	Occurrence is sporadic; only a proportion of affected birds die	On morphology and location of this nematode	None

KEY

AC	allantoic cavity	ELISA	enzyme-linked immunosorbent assay
AGP	agar gel precipitation	EM	electron microscopy
AF	allantoic fluid	GI	growth inhibition
CAM	chorioallantoic membrane	IF	immunofluorescence
		HA	haemagglutination
		HI	haemagglutination inhibition
		RSA	rapid slide agglutination
		SN	serum neutralization
		TA	tube agglutination

several weeks or months in empty buildings. They can also use wild birds as reservoir hosts so that mite infestations remain an ongoing major problem.

MITES

These include the pathogenically more serious "red mite" (*Dermanyssus gallinae*) (Fig. 5.5), its relative the "northern fowl mite" (*Ornithonyssus = Liponyssus sylviarum*) (Fig. 5.6), and the less common burrowing mite *Knemidocoptes* (= *Cnemidocoptes*). The two surface dwelling mites can be very harmful and individual populations of *Dermanyssus* may exceed 250 000, virtually exsanguinating the host which may die with a terminal haematocrit level as low as 4 per cent. *Dermanyssus* and *Ornithonyssus* have different types of life cycle: *Dermanyssus* feeds mainly in the middle of the night, quitting the bird to lay its eggs, so that sizeable infestations may be missed during a day-time inspection of the host. *Ornithonyssus* remain on the host permanently.

Adult red mites resemble red, black or grey dots depending on when they last fed; they can complete their life cycle in

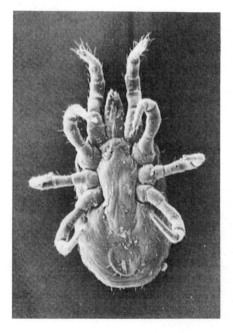

Fig. 5.5
Dermanyssus gallinae (red mite).

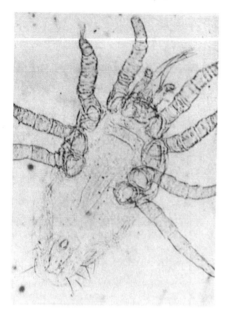

Fig. 5.6
Ornithonyssus (= Liponyssus) sylviarum
(northern fowl mite).

only one week and fed female mites can then starve for 6–9 months. Eggs are laid 12–24 h after the feed and hatch within 48–72 h. Although chickens are the usual host, pigeons, turkeys, canaries, budgerigars and wild birds are equally susceptible, and red mites will migrate to the upper rooms of houses and hospitals from birds' nests in the eaves of the roof. The resting and oviposition sites favoured by replete red mites include such surprising microhabitats as cross-over points in apparently clean wire cages and the slotted ends of cage bird perches, as well as cracks in walls and floors.

Ornithonyssus sylviarum is probably the most important external parasite of chickens in temperate areas of the world. It is also seen more often than *Dermanyssus* since it breeds continuously on the host. Eggs are laid mainly around the cooler region; the mites then tend to move to the neck, leaving the vent area looking dirty with a heavy contamination of mite eggs and excreta. Like *Dermanyssus*, *Ornithonyssus* can complete its life cycle in less than one week under suitably warm conditions but fed mites survive for only 3–4 weeks. Individual birds vary in their susceptibility to *Ornithonyssus*, some harbouring very large numbers, others hardly any at all. Differential diagnosis of the two genera of mites is important because of their egg-laying habits and resting sites, which obviously require different approaches to control. Apart from blood in their gut caeca, *Dermanyssus* will also show microscopically a characteristic triangular ventral anal plate, compared with the pear-drop plate of *Ornithonyssus*. The mouthparts of *Dermanyssus* are also long, wiry and protusible, while those of *Ornithonyssus* are short and end in tiny pincers.

There are three species of *Knemidocoptes*: *K. gallinae* (depluming itch mite) (Fig. 5.7), *K. mutans* (scaly leg mite) (Figs 5.8 and 5.9) and *K. pilae* (scaly beak mite of budgerigars). The depluming mite is the most important; it can cause feather loss, stimulating cannibalistic behaviour by other birds. The scaly leg mite lives under the scales of the legs; this is normally a "backyard" problem in older stock but can be a serious nuisance, showing as irritable lesions covered with white flakes and powder. *K. pilae* attacks the edge of the beak and may cause unsightly horny outgrowths in this area. *Knemidocoptes* is diagnosed by removing a small portion of scale and warming it on a slide in 10 per cent potassium or sodium hydroxide; this visualizes the 170–500 µm stumpy legged mites in the skin material.

Suitable acaricides include dusts or sprays of the organophosphorus compounds malathion, diazinon, tetrachlorvinphos, dichlorvos or tetrachlorvinphos or the carbamate carbaryl. Plastic strips incorporating pyrethroids such as permethrin have given good mite control in caged birds in the US for up to one year.

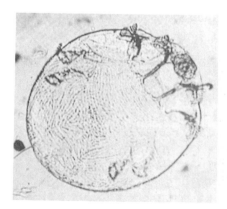

Fig. 5.7
Knemidocoptes gallinae.

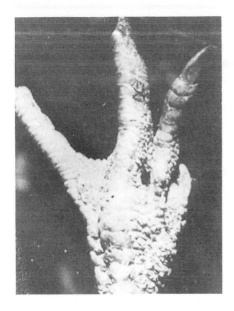

Fig. 5.8
Scaly leg lesions (*Knemidocoptes mutans*).

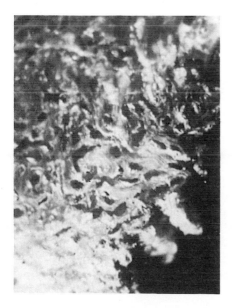

Fig. 5.9
Tunnels made by the mite *Knemidocoptes mutans* (scaly leg).

LICE

All bird lice are of the chewing (biting) type so that none can cause anaemia—they all produce their parasitic effects by feeding on the feathers or skin, causing considerable irritation. It is possible that heavy infestations of lice really do make the host feel "lousy", perhaps due to toxic material entering the system. Individual birds may harbour several species of lice at the same time.

The most common chicken lice are *Menacanthus stramineus* (body louse), *Menopon gallinae* (shaft louse) and *L. caponis* (wing louse); *Goniocotes, Goniodes* and *Lipeurus* may also occur on poultry. Turkeys may share *M. stramineus* with chickens, while ducks and gees may harbour *Anaticola*. Individual birds can support large numbers of lice, although older birds tend to suffer far less from these parasites than chicks, which may even succumb to pediculosis.

Lousiness is preventable if care is taken to introduce only clean birds into louse-free houses, and infestations from wild birds should never occur in modern husbandry practice. Louse numbers tend to rise during the cooler months, so that poultry flocks should be checked for lice and treated before the onset of colder weather. Floor birds are most easily treated by applying 4–5 per cent dusts of organophosphorus insecticides such as malathion or carbaryl. Severe louse infestations on caged birds can be controlled by placing malathion dust boxes in the cages. For complete control, floor treatment can be repeated after four weeks and direct bird treatment after two weeks. Some poultrymen recommend the application of a high pressure spray of insecticide to the entire interior of the house including birds; 2 per cent malathion is very effective for this purpose.

FLEAS

Only *Ceratophyllus gallinae* is likely to be found on poultry in Britain; it breeds in any "filling" including the wall insulation and roof space of the poultry house. Like the red mite, fed female fleas can survive for several months after a blood meal. Malathion sprays are again very safe and effective, and new litter should be treated with this insecticide if fleas have been a problem.

As with all the parasites mentioned, good husbandry and cleanliness are half the battle, and the application of insecticide aerosols, sprays or dusts wastes time and money if conditions of the poultry house continue to favour a build up of parasites.

ACKNOWLEDGEMENTS

Our thanks are due to Dr F. T. W. Jordan for helpful comments.

REFERENCES AND FURTHER READING

Gregory, M. W. & Norton, C. C. (1986) *Veterinary Record* Supplement *In Practice* **8**, 33.

Hofstad, M. S. (1984) (ed.) *Diseases of Poultry*, 8th edn. Ames, Iowa, Iowa State University Press.

Schofield, A. M. (1983) *A Checklist of the Helminth Parasites of Domestic Animals of the United Kingdom*. Milton Keynes, Hoechst UK Ltd.

Soulsby, E. J. L. (1982) *Helminths, Arthropods and Protozoa of Domesticated Animals*, 7th edn. London, Baillière Tindall.

CHAPTER 6

Vaccination Regimes for Poultry

DON HAXBY

INTRODUCTION

Certain regimes of vaccination for domestic poultry concentrating on (1) breeders with special reference to commercial layer parent, broiler parent and turkey parent stock; (2) commercial laying stock; (3) broilers and (4) fattening turkeys are presented. The regimes must be considered as entirely basic and must be adjusted according to the immunological state of the recipient birds and current disease problems, international, national and local.

Grandparent and parent breeding stock constitute the genetic input into the whole breeding operation and are therefore valuable and subject to an intensive vaccination programme in the interests of animal health, protection of the offspring, production and welfare. Longevity is naturally also of great importance.

Poultry do not differ from any other species of domestic animal in that maternal antibody is transferred to the offspring but, in the case of poultry, this occurs through the egg. In some cases the antibody present in the newly hatched chick dictates the vaccination programme recommended.

Maternal antibody recedes quite rapidly, having a half-life of approximately four-and-a-half days in the laying bird, but tends to decay more quickly in the broiler because of its accelerated growth rate. It usually becomes exhausted by 21 days. However, it can linger for considerable periods of time, where oil-based vaccines have been used in the parent bird. This is particularly important with Gumboro disease, where the original Gumboro disease spray vaccine will not be effective in the presence of maternal antibody. Some viruses can overcome moderate levels of maternal antibody in which case 21 days is generally accepted as a reasonable time to commence vaccination.

Another consideration is that chickens may be subjected in early life to infectious bursitis (infectious bursal disease or Gumboro disease) which has an immunosuppressive effect due to destruction of the bursa of Fabricius and its functions. Such birds have a lowered resistance to disease and equally manifest a negative or suboptimal response to vaccines.

BASIC CONSIDERATIONS

As with all vaccination techniques and, more especially, where live vaccines are used, certain fundamental criteria must be observed:

(1)   Only healthy stock should be vaccinated.
(2)   Administration of the vaccine must be carried out in accordance with the recommendations contained in the data sheet.
(3)   Vaccine storage recommendations (usually between 2 and 8°C) and reconstitution procedures should be strictly adhered to and any unused vaccine discarded in accordance with the current health and safety regulations and COSHH provisions. Any freeze-dried vaccine, once reconstituted, should be used immediately following the withholding of water from the birds as recommended on the vaccine data sheet. This route of administration is commonly used in poultry flocks.

COSHH regulations. In Britain, the Control of Substances Hazardous to Health (COSHH) Regulations require that all vaccine that remains unused at the end of a vaccination session should be mixed with an approved disinfectant and time be allowed for inactivation before it is discarded. All containers should be disposed of to a landfill site via an approved waste disposal contractor.

(4) It is essential that when in-water vaccination is used, the vaccine should be mixed with a human skimmed milk product to protect it against chlorine and heavy metal ions which inactivate live vaccines. Poultry producers have tried using calf and sheep milk products which are high in fat; when this occurs the fat globules tend to bind up the vaccine virus removing it from the system and thereby reducing the concentration of the vaccine administered to the birds. A recommended skimmed milk inclusion rate is 500 ml of skimmed milk to 7.5 litres (2 gallons) of water. The water source should be clean and free from detergent and disinfectant residues.

Drinking water vaccination is really only suitable for birds of over two weeks of age. When using this technique one must ensure that all vaccine medicated water is consumed within 2 h of the vaccine being added. Sufficient containers should be available to ensure that adequate drinking space is accessible to all the birds. Water deprivation to stimulate thirst would normally be necessary: the length of time required depending on the ambient temperature and the type of bird being vaccinated. Vaccination should always be done in the early morning and in sunny weather always protect the vaccine and vaccine medicated water from direct sunlight.

The approximate number of gallons of water required to vaccinate a flock varies with age as follows:

2 weeks	2 gallons/1000 birds	9 08
3 weeks	3 gallons/1000 birds	13.62
4 weeks	4 gallons/1000 birds	18.16

(5) Spray vaccination is also commonly used in intensive poultry operations and the aerosol dispersion is best achieved by using 500 ml of diluent (distilled water) for 1000 birds. The cloud of particles should become invisible not less than 3 m from the aerosol machine. Most machines are adjustable. Normally coarse sprays are used in young chicks at day old and 3 weeks while fine sprays are used in older birds that have received a priming vaccination earlier in the rearing period. Where coarse sprays are used it is important that the lighting is turned up high after the vaccine has been administered to encourage the birds to "peck" the droplets

of vaccine. With fine sprays it is important that the ventilation is severely reduced during vaccination administration so that the fine aerosol particles are not desiccated, thus reducing the effectiveness of the vaccine.

It is important that respiratory protective equipment is used by all personnel who administer or are present at the use of vaccines using spray administration techniques.

(6)   Other methods of vaccine administration are also commonly practised. Injection techniques are used for vaccination against Marek's disease, Newcastle disease, paramyxo disease in pigeons, infectious bronchitis, Gumboro disease, *Pasteurella* and erysipelas infections. In addition, "eyedrop" instillation is used against infectious bronchitis and infectious laryngitis, the "wing stab" or feather follicle method for fowl pox vaccines and "foot web stab" method for duck virus hepatitis.

(7)   Flock, site and vaccination histories of the birds being presented for vaccination are of great value in determining the programme to be followed, as also is the current disease situation in the country, area or immediate locality.

Table 6.1 Breeders (commercial layer parent and broiler parent).

Age	Vaccine	Dose	Route of administration
Day-old	Marek's disease	1:1	By injection
3 weeks	Live infectious bronchitis + live Newcastle disease + live intermediate Gumboro vaccine (optional)	1:1	In drinking water
or 4 weeks	As 3 weeks + live Gumboro	1:1	In drinking water
or 3 + 4 weeks	Live intermediate Gumboro vaccine	1:1	In drinking water
7 weeks	Live Newcastle disease + live Gumboro vaccine	1:1	In drinking water or aerosol
10 weeks	Live Gumboro vaccine (if birds have not seroconverted)	1:1	In drinking water or aerosol
12 weeks	Epidemic tremor	1:1	In drinking water
16 weeks	Inactivated Newcastle	1:1	By injection
	Gumboro disease,	1:1	By injection
	infectious bronchitis	1:1	By injection

Table 6.2 Commercial layers.

Age	Vaccine	Dose	Route of administration
Day-old	Marek's disease,	1:1	By injection
	live infectious bronchitis	1:1	By coarse spray
Day-old	Inactivated Gumboro (optional)	1:1	By injection
3 weeks	Combined live infectious bronchitis + live Newcastle disease,	1:1	By spray
	live intermediate Gumboro if not given inactivated at day-old	1:1	In drinking water
4 weeks	Live Gumboro if not given inactivated at day-old	1:1	In drinking water
5 weeks	Live intermediate Gumboro if not inactivated at day-old	1:1	In drinking water
9 weeks	Live infectious bronchitis + live Newcastle combined	1:1	In drinking water
12 weeks	Epidemic tremor	1:1	In drinking water
16 weeks	Inactivated Newcastle,	1:1	By injection
	infectious bronchitis,	1:1	By injection
	Egg drop syndrome 76,	1:1	By injection
	Gumboro disease (inactivated) (optional)	1:1	By injection

Table 6.3 Coccidiosis vaccine.

Used in commercial layers and broiler breeders in rearing at 7–10 days of age
Live attenuated precocious strains of *Eimeria* at a dose rate of 1:1 via drinking water

(8) Other considerations to be taken into account are the welfare and economic significance of the disease, the efficacy of the vaccines available, possible side effects of the chosen vaccine plus the costs and labour necessary to carry out the vaccination.

(9) Precautions should be taken when using any oil-based injectable vaccines so that the operator does not administer

Table 6.4 Broilers.

Age	Vaccine	Dose	Route of administration
Day-old	Live infectious bronchitis at hatchery,	1:1	Coarse Spray/ Eye Drops
	Marek's disease (if the birds are intended for the heavy broilers trade)	1:1	By injection
17 days	Live Gumboro intermediate disease (optional)	1:1	In drinking water
25 days	Live intermediate Gumboro disease (optional),	1:1	In drinking water
	live infectious bronchitis (if birds growing on)	1:1	In drinking water
30 days	Live intermediate Gumboro disease (optional) depending on infection history on premises	1:1	In drinking water

Table 6.5 Turkey breeders.

Age	Vaccine	Dose	Route of administration
0–7 days	Live attenuated TRT*	1:1	Spray
5 weeks	Live (Newcastle)	1:1	Spray
8–9 weeks	Live (Newcastle)	1:1	Spray
11–12 weeks	*Pasteurella*/erysipelas vaccine + inactivated Newcastle	1:1	Injection
12 weeks	Live attenuated TRT	1:1	Injection
16–20 weeks	*Pasteurella*/erysipelas vaccine	1:1	Injection
25–28 weeks	*Pasteurella*/erysipelas vaccine + inactivated Newcastle + killed TRT	1:1	Injection

*Turkey rhinotracheitis (TRT).

the vaccine to him or herself. If this happens it should be treated as a medical emergency. Advice should be sought immediately to avoid a very painful reaction occasioned by the adjuvant and limit possible complications. It is wise to take the data sheet for the product which has been accidentally injected to the general practitioner or hospital.

Table 6.6 Fattening turkeys.

Live Newcastle 1:1 by spray at least twice, preferably three times
Erysipelas/*Pasteurella* depending on flock history, this being important
 with turkeys reared on farms for the Christmas trade
Fattening turkeys are all routinely vaccinated with live attenuated TRT. *It
 should be stressed that this product is no longer licensed for multi age sites
 due to severe reactions and complications.* Most usage is 0–7 days by
 spray.

VACCINATION PROGRAMMES

The regimes shown in Tables 6.1–6.6 may be considered as standard but obviously they may be varied according to the diseases current at the time. Equally, the method of administration changes in accordance with the husbandry methods used.

The programmes listed are designed for large units but may be adapted for smaller units and backyard flocks. However, it should be remembered that few of the vaccines recommended are available in small quantities. Three special vaccines for pigeons are available: one contains the pigeon paramyxo virus specifically while the others are based on chicken Newcastle virus; one contains a synthetic adjuvant, the other two are oil based.

Most of the vaccines used can be monitored serologically to detect the level of antibody achieved, and indications for revaccination established, where vaccinal response is low or negative.

I would suggest that if in any doubt over vaccines, vaccination techniques and administration that you should contact any of the major manufacturers who have veterinary advisers who would be only to willing to give advice.

ACKNOWLEDGEMENTS

The author wishes to acknowledge with grateful thanks, the advice and help so willingly and freely given to him by Dr Ann-Marie Farmer, BVSc, DVBiol, PhD, MRCVS, and Stephen A. Lister, BSc, BVetMed, MRCVS.

CHAPTER 7

Common Diseases in Turkeys Reared for the Christmas Market

IAN MACPHERSON

INTRODUCTION

In order to provide advice on preventive medication and treatment of a turkey flock, the veterinary surgeon should have sufficient background information of the farm rearing facilities (Fig. 7.1) and a history of the flock. Should disease occur, a representative sample of birds must be submitted for post mortem examination.

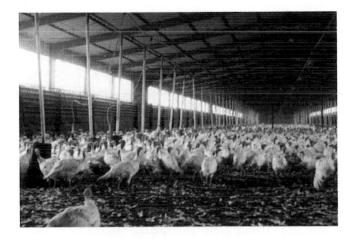

Fig. 7.1
Typical housing of
turkeys in a pole
barn.

ARRIVAL OF POULTS

Before poults even arrive, the house, feeders and drinkers should be thoroughly cleaned and disinfected and the floor covered with new wood shavings. Clean mains water in suitably designed drinkers plus a specific turkey starter diet are necessary for successful rearing.

A bright tungsten light (100 W) suspended over shallow feed pans or apple trays and drinkers on the floor close by the feed area will encourage immediate feeding. One feeder or drinker should be available per 20 or 30 poults. Radiant gas brooders provide the best heating and can be adjusted by height or temperature control so that a temperature of 95°F (35°C) is achieved at turkey level for the first 24 hours. This can be progressively reduced to a rearing fattening temperature for uncontrolled environment facilities of 50–55°F (10–12.5°C). A 1°F reduction per day, together with close monitoring of the bird behaviour and ambient temperature, will ensure that gas brooding can stop (except in the cold evenings) by the time the birds are five to six weeks old when they should be well covered with feathers. Poults received late in the afternoon should be fed and watered immediately. They are then best left in darkness to rest for 12–14 h to recover from hatching, sexing and the trauma of transportation. Up to 20 h of light may be provided in the first few days of life to encourage feeding but by the time the birds are 7–10 days old, day length should be maintained at no more than 14 h for the fattening period. Light intensity should be of the order of 5–10 lux at bird level. It is quite possible for birds to see and find food and water at much lower intensities, e.g. 0.5 lux.

These procedures should cut down mortality due to "starve out" syndrome or to non-starters that are failing to find food and water. Losses in the first week should be of the order of 1–2 per cent.

Beak trimming to prevent cannibalism is generally carried out at one week old. Occasionally mortality can occur due to rough handling and infection; sometimes poults will haemorrhage heavily after trimming for no apparent reason. Prevention of overheating plus supplementation with vitamins and vitamin K analogues will help minimize losses.

IMPORTANT DISEASES IN THE FIRST TWO WEEKS OF LIFE

YOLK SAC INFECTION (OMPHALITIS)

Infection of the yolk sac (sometimes known as navel infection) can be a major cause of mortality in the first five days of life. It is generally a manifestation of imperfect hatching egg hygiene or poor practice in the hatchery. Poults are found dead with swollen abdomens and food in the gizzard and intestine. The yolk sac is frequently dark red and it has an unpleasant fetid odour. Bacterial examination may reveal a profusion of organisms including *Escherichia coli*, *Bacillus cereus*, enterococci, pseudomonas and sometimes clostridia and proteus. Death probably results from toxaemia or septicaemia.

Birds with a subacute yolk sac infection frequently survive but remain slow growers. Infection is not contagious and the affected birds are best culled out. Additional heat and vitamin supplement in drinking water for three to four days may be of some value.

"STARVE OUT" (Fig. 7.2)

Yolk sac infection is easily distinguished from a "starve out" where yolk sacs are normally absorbed but no food is found within the intestine or the gizzard. The liver is usually a yellowish bronze colour with a prominent gall bladder. Here the bird has simply died from malnutrition because it cannot find food, some other condition has induced inappetence or because of some physical abnormality such as blindness or cross beak. Urates in the kidney indicate lack of water.

ASPERGILLOSIS

Aspergillosis, caused by the fungus *Aspergillus* species, is frequently seen in individual cases of death in older turkeys where respiratory problems are evident. However, it can be seen in the first week or two of life as an acute disease affecting a high proportion of the flock with a resultant mortality of 10–20 per cent. In young poults extensive

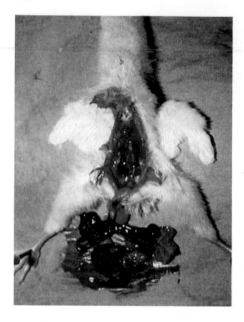

Fig. 7.2
Case of starve out in a turkey poult

aspergillosis can result from a hatchery infection and affect birds in the first 48 h of life. Affected poults gasp and breathe rapidly through the open beak (without respiratory rales). There is not usually any ocular or nasal discharge.

Examination of young poult carcases will reveal pinhead yellow nodules in the lungs and air sacs (Fig. 7.3). In older turkeys these will often be quite large and white with green

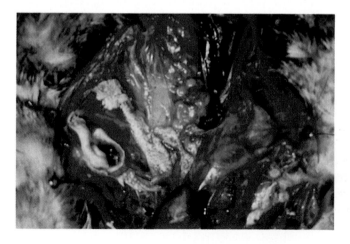

Fig. 7.3
Case of turkey aspergillosis shows pinhead yellow nodules in the lungs and air sacs.

centres, producing plaque-like lesions on the air sac walls throughout the abdominal area as well as the thoracic areas. Incision of the lungs will frequently show caseous nodules embedded within lung tissue.

Presumptive diagnosis can be made upon the lesions found, confirmation depending on microscopic examination and fungus culture. Signs of respiratory distress in older turkeys in which aspergillosis is involved may frequently be caused by contamination of the environment through large numbers of spores in the litter or food. These can be related to high humidity owing to poor ventilation.

There is no satisfactory treatment for aspergillosis in turkeys and, in the case of very young poults, those affected are best destroyed. In adult birds it is not generally a flock problem and individuals can be culled out. Quaternary ammonium disinfectants at 0.01 per cent concentration in the drinking water appear to help.

CLINICAL SALMONELLOSIS

Salmonella pullorum or *S. gallinarum* are not likely to be present in turkeys received from commercial hatcheries. However, mortality can occasionally occur in the first week of life owing to infection with other salmonellas and, in particular, *Salmonella typhimurium*. This infection may either be egg transmitted or picked up in the environment of the rearing and brooding facility.

No specific signs will usually be observed other than increased mortality and occasionally blindness. Some birds may have yolk sac infection and cores of pus in the caeca.

Direct and indirect culture from yolk sac or liver will produce non-lactose fermenting bacteria which need further laboratory examination to confirm the organism involved. Treatment is generally of little value and is not to be recommended as antibiotics are likely to create chronic carriers of infection. Should it appear that the disease is affecting the flock as a whole, then in order to prevent mortality and reduce suffering in the poults, treatment with furazolidone in the food at a concentration of 0.02 per cent for 10 days is highly effective in controlling mortality. Alternatively furaltadone may be given via the drinking water at a concentration of

0.02 per cent. However, turkeys are extremely susceptible to nitrofuran poisoning and this treatment should be exercised with care and higher levels avoided in birds less than two weeks old.

CARDIOHEPATIC SYNDROME (OEDEMA DISEASE)

Cardiohepatic syndrome was first reported in the UK in 1968. It generally affects male poults growing strongly between 4 and 20 days of age, the most common age being 10–14 days. The cause of this condition has not been established but it does not appear to be infectious and is probably caused by poor management such as overcrowding, overheating or disinfectant fumes. It is most common in late summer months when poult hatching is at its peak.

The faster growing and biggest poults are usually found dead. Mortality will usually be between 1 and 5 per cent, but occasionally 20 per cent has been seen. In uncomplicated outbreaks losses will continue over a 5–10 day period.

Affected poults have a noticeably enlarged abdomen which contains clear or slightly bloodstained fluid. The liver is swollen and curved with rounded edges (Fig. 7.4). On

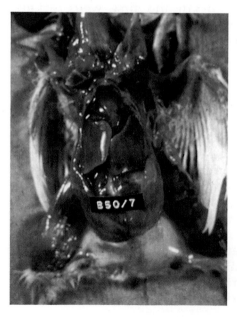

Fig. 7.4
Oedema disease in turkey poult. Note swollen and curved liver with rounded edges.

palpation it is usually harder than normal and the gall bladder is often distended. In more chronic cases the heart can be distended and the artery and great veins dilated. The kidneys are usually very swollen and have fine urate deposits on the surface. Carcase fat is usually pink and intestinal blood vessels, especially in the duodenal area, are dilated. The general appearance of the musculature of the carcase is moist and oedematous. In the more chronic cases appearing at 4–6 weeks old the principal lesion is a grossly dilated rounded flabby heart with a yellow brown shrunken liver and no ascites.

No particular treatment is available and supportive therapy such as multivitamins and electrolytes is of little value.

DISEASES OF THE POST BROODING PERIOD—ENTERIC

COCCIDIOSIS

Of the nine known *Eimeria* species reported in the turkey, probably only four or five are of importance, particularly in semi-intensive conditions.

Eimeria adenoides can be highly pathogenic in young turkeys of 2–4 weeks of age and parasitizes the lower small intestine and caeca. After about 5 or 6 weeks old it does not appear to cause disease. Affected birds have thick white mucoid exudate, often with casts and caecal plugs in the lower intestine and rectal area. Smears will demonstrate numerous oocysts and gametocytes at the site of infection.

E. meleagrimitis can also affect young turkeys causing mortality around 4–6 weeks of age. Lesions are found in the duodenum and jejunum of the upper intestine. There are often haemorrhagic streaks in the wall of the intestine together with a mucoid exudate which contains numerous oocysts and gametocytes. *E. meleagridis* infects the caecum and lower ileum and rectum giving rise to the caecal cores in which oocysts are found. Clinical signs are rare but birds may be submitted for reasons of unthriftiness or poor weight gain.

Turkeys appear to become resistant to coccidial infection from about 10 weeks old. Infections have been very occasionally recorded in much older birds. Under practical farming conditions this is not likely to be a problem and it is usually economically prudent to stop using coccidiostats in the feed at about 10 weeks old.

An infected flock should be treated with a combination of amprolium and ethopabate in the drinking water, possibly for up to 10 days, strictly in accord with the manufacturer's recommendations.

The disease is less prevalent today in both modern intensive systems and turkeys reared under semi-intensive conditions for the Christmas market. This is largely due to the provision of more effective coccidiostats such as the ionophores monensin sodium and lasalocid sodium. In addition to these compounds halofuginone, clopidol, a combination of clopidol and methyl benzoquate or amprolium, sulphaquinoxaline and ethopabate provide effective prevention against coccidiosis in the turkey poult.

Some fear has been expressed regarding the use of ionophores in turkeys but provided the manufacturer's recommended levels are adhered to and the drug is administered continuously from day old up to 8–16 weeks of age, or 5 days before slaughter, there are no problems. However, problems can arise where ionophores are suddenly introduced to turkeys at six weeks old or more, which have never been previously exposed to ionophore medication. Should this happen the signs are quite typical: excitement followed by paralysis with head and legs extended. Often the triangular abductor muscle on the interior aspect of the thigh may be much paler than the surrounding flesh and occasional lesions may also be seen in the myocardium. Complete diagnosis can be effected by the history of the food given to the birds and, if available, analysis of that food.

Treatment consists of removing the offending feed and assisting the paralysed birds to reach water. Recovery is often seen without any sequelae within 24 h in those birds which have not consumed too high a dose of the drug; otherwise mortality may continue to occur for 3–4 days after the removal of the food.

It must be emphasized that this type of finding is very uncommon and generally associated with abuse or malpractice in the use of ionophores in turkeys. The two ionophores salinomycin sodium and narasin do not have product licences for turkeys and should not under present circumstances be prescribed for use in this species. The use of tiamulin is contraindicated in the presence of ionophorous compounds.

HISTOMONIASIS

Histomoniasis was at one time very common in turkeys. It also affects chickens, pheasants and partridges. Species should not be run together because of the risks of cross infection through the intermediate host, the caecal worm *Hetarakis gallinarum*. Eggs from the latter are infected with histomonads and the disease can lie dormant in fold yards or crevices in concreted areas for long periods of time and then reappear.

Infection is usually initiated after ingestion of embryonated eggs of *H. gallinarum* from food, soil or litter contaminated with faecal material. The protozoan parasites contained within the larvae of *H. gallinarum* are released in the caeca a few days later. During this phase of multiplication there is little or no pathological change. After about seven days necrosis of the caecal tissue takes place and by the 10th day lesions begin to apear in the liver. These become large and numerous 2–3 weeks after infection.

Poults generally will have lost appetite and shown signs of watery diarrhoea with deaths occurring 10–12 days after infection. On post mortem examination the caeca are seen to be grossly enlarged and contain large cores of necrotic material (Fig. 7.5). Liver lesions are conspicuous, being circular and cream coloured necrotic masses on the surface of the liver which extend into the parenchyma. Mortality in untreated and unmedicated flocks can be as high as 80 per cent.

In modern turkey feeds medication for the prevention of histomoniasis is generally practised using dimetridazole. Dimetridazole can also be used for treatment in the food or drinking water. Control of the disease is difficult due to the prolonged time in which infected *Hetarakis* eggs will survive. If infection has become established on a turkey unit, particularly with earth floors, assume that it will perpetuate and preventive medication will always be required.

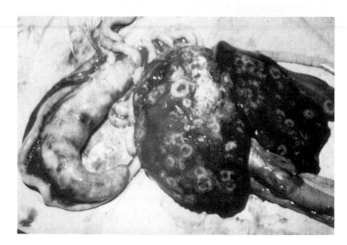

Fig. 7.5
Liver and caeca from
a case of
histomoniasis with
cream coloured
necrotic masses on
the liver surface and
gross enlargement of
the caeca.

HAEMORRHAGIC ENTERITIS

Haemorrhagic enteritis is caused by an adenovirus analogous to the causal agent of marble spleen disease in pheasants. The culture and isolation of these particular viruses is very difficult and has only recently been successfully achieved. Antibody to haemorrhagic enteritis of turkeys is widespread in breeding flocks and fattening birds over 13 or 14 weeks of age. It is likely that the young poult is protected by maternal antibody for the first 4–5 weeks of life. The disease is unusual in birds under five weeks of age and the most common age for the onset of disease is between eight and 12 weeks. The signs may be sudden with deaths occurring within 24 h. Dark red staining of the feathers of the vent area and bloody diarrhoea can be seen in affected birds.

Birds lose a large quantity of blood into the intestine so that on death they appear to have a pale anaemic head. Once the disease has occurred in the flock recovery takes about two weeks. Birds are refractory to reinfection but may suffer from immunosuppression and be susceptible to other diseases.

Post mortem examination may reveal distended intestines with dark blood stained mucus and food with occasional necrotic areas, especially in the duodenum and anterior small intestine. Liver, kidney and spleen are swollen and sometimes haemorrhagic. Incision of the spleen shows a marbled appearance due to the enlarged and prominent white pulp areas. In less acute outbreaks a mucoid enteritis may be the only lesion seen, with the birds passing dark tarry faeces. The spleen will be enlarged and marbled, even though the other organs appear normal. It is possible to demonstrate intranuclear inclusion bodies of the adenovirus in the spleen and duodenal mucosa.

Treatment should be aimed at minimizing the effect of secondary bacteria using non-absorbable antibiotics, for example, neomycin. If secondary colisepticaemia is suspected treatment with nitrofurones or tetracyclines together with electrolytes and vitamins as supportive therapy will assist in recovery from dehydration and septicaemia.

In the UK at present there are no licensed vaccines for the prevention of this disease but in the USA and France avirulent strains of the virus derived from harvested spleen have been used for prevention.

RESPIRATORY DISEASES OF THE POST BROODING PERIOD

COLISEPTICAEMIA

Escherichia coli infection in turkey poults is primarily a septicaemic disease with infection involving the upper respiratory tract and air sacs of the thoracic and abdominal region. The first signs of infection often follow stress or chilling, particularly when associated with damp litter and poor ventilation. An increase in daily mortality will often be the first indication of an outbreak of colisepticaemia without the flock as a whole developing rales or snicking. The latter, however, may be audible in the dark when the flock is silent and on occasions harsh coughing will be heard. Affected birds will be listless and the flock's food consumption reduced. Several birds can be found dead one day, then mortality apparently ceases for one or two days until another batch of birds will be found dead. Affected birds appear hunch backed and miserable and frequently have dirty ruffled feathers and diarrhoea.

Diagnosis can be made upon the history and clinical signs together with the almost pathognomonic lesions of congested

carcase, dark swollen liver often showing surface haemorrhages (Fig. 7.6) and the isolation of *E. coli*. Pericarditis and
perihepatitis, which is frequently characteristic of broiler
colisepticaemia, is not often present in turkeys. In its place
can be seen an exudative air sacculitis particularly if there
are associated infections of viral or mycoplasma origin. If
respiratory signs are severe in turkeys then consideration
must be given to the presence of contagious or notifiable
virus disease such as Newcastle disease or fowl plague.

Treatment involves the use of antibiotics and other drugs
to which the *E. coli* is sensitive. Effective treatment is generally
provided by immediate administration in the drinking water
of a broad spectrum antibiotic such as chlortetracycline,
oxytetracycline or furaltadone.

Alleviation of the major signs may be achieved by water
medication but occasionally it may be necessary to follow this
five or six day period of treatment with in-feed medication
using either nitrofurans at 0.02–0.04 per cent or tetracyclines
at 200–300 g per ton for 2–3 weeks.

ALCALIGENES TRACHEITIS (Fig. 7.7)

Alcaligenes tracheitis can follow the onset of haemorrhagic
enteritis, which may be a precipitating factor, affecting birds
from 4 to 10 weeks of age. The causal agent is *Alcaligenes
faecalis*. In an affected flock turkey poults show respiratory

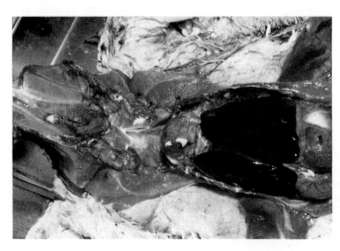

Fig. 7.6
Congested carcase
of turkey with *E. coli*
septicaemia, showing
dark swollen liver.

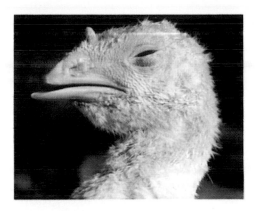

Fig. 7.7
Bird with alcaligenes tracheitis.

rales and increased nasal discharge, frequently with a foamy conjunctivitis.

Flocks, particularly males, may produce a high-pitched rasping sound instead of the normal gobble. Respiratory signs last for approximately two weeks. In uncomplicated cases the lesions are confined to the trachea which contains excessive amounts of mucoid exudate, but not haemorrhagic material, and in contrast air sacs and lungs appear normal. To confirm diagnosis, the isolation of *A. faecalis* is required. The differential diagnosis or implication of complicating factors such as viruses, secondary bacteria and mycoplasma as well as environmental mismanagement need to be taken into consideration.

Treatment of affected flocks, other than to minimize further infection, has not been very successful, even though *A. faecalis* is susceptible *in vitro* to many of the Gram-negative and broad spectrum antibiotics. Only spectinomycin appears to be satisfactory in treating the disease.

Control relies upon good hygiene and husbandry, prevention of overcrowding and stress factors and, in particular, providing supplies of clean water. The sheds should be properly disinfected following the infection.

RHINOTRACHEITIS

Turkey rhinotracheitis was first reported in the UK in 1985. It is thought to be viral in origin, but frequently associated bacteria include *E. coli*, *Moraxella antipestifer*, *Bordetella*-like species and *Pseudomonas* species. Research in France since 1981 has shown a number of common viruses to be present in outbreaks but not apparently associated with the disease. These include paramyxoviruses, avian influenza virus and reovirus. Recent studies in this country and France have pointed to different virus types as being the main causal agent, notably adenovirus, coronavirus, orthomyxovirus or an embryo lethal virus.

Circumstantial evidence from the field indicates vertical transmission from affected parent flocks, as well as droplet spread. Clinical signs can be seen in birds as young as 10 days old but more commonly in the 3–5 week age group. Rearing turkeys and flocks in lay have also succumbed to the disease. The latter had severe falls in egg production over 1–2 weeks with recovery over a further 2–3 week period. Egg shell quality and colour are markedly affected together with reduced hatchability and an increase in second quality poults.

Clinical signs in the young poults are of acute respiratory distress with a high-pitched cough and nasal discharge or a very mild and almost inapparent respiratory syndrome. Morbidity is almost 100 per cent and mortality from 1 to 30 per cent. Deaths in young birds follow a severe rhinitis with copious ocular and nasal discharge, sinusitis and a mucoid tracheitis. The trachea can become occluded by mucous or caseous plugs causing death. Secondary infections with *E. coli, Moraxella* or *Bordetella* species and *Pseudomonas* types are common. A secondary wave of mortality can often occur some 3–4 weeks later with secondary bacteria being involved with an upsurge of air sacculitis and septicaemia. This may be a result of a possible immunosuppression following the initial infection or a concomitant haemorrhagic septicaemia.

Post mortem examination reveals a sinusitis, mucopurulent tracheitis and possibly air sacculitis and splenomegaly.

Recovery takes place slowly and is dependent upon management and stress factors such as stocking density and ventilation rates. Treatment with antibiotics and vitamins is generally of little value and careful husbandry is required to minimize the effects of the disease. Frequently condemnations due to air sacculitis are much higher on inspection than the clinical appearance of a recovered flock would indicate.

FOWL CHOLERA (AVIAN PASTEURELLOSIS)

Fowl cholera is a contagious disease affecting both domesticated and wild birds and generally appears as a septicaemia or pneumonia associated with high morbidity and mortality.

Strains of *Pasteurella multocida* may vary in virulence and pathogenicity. A variety of factors precipitate the disease, in particular stress and the incidence of vectors such as rats and mice. The organism does not survive well outside the body and is susceptible to disinfectants and general good hygiene practices. Turkeys appear to be more susceptible than any other domestic fowl, except possibly waterfowl.

The disease is generally observed in turkeys in the peracute or acute form. In the former there may be no initial signs and large numbers of birds in the flock are suddenly found dead but in good bodily condition. The acute form shows marked depression, anorexia, cyanosis, oral sanguineous discharges and fetid diarrhoea. In some chronic cases, lameness and torticollis may develop.

Post mortem examination lesions include congestion of the carcase with multiple petechiation throughout the viscera and pinpoint necrotic foci in the liver. The lungs are frequently pneumonic and have a characteristic cooked meat appearance. Perihepatitis may occur.

Culture of the causal organism will confirm the disease and in peracute cases impression smears of the liver or heart stained with methylene blue will show bipolar staining organisms.

Peracute cholera is so rapid in onset that treatment is of little value. In the more common acute and subacute forms drugs have proved to be effective so long as medication continues. Treatment includes sulphaquinoxaline or sulphamethazine in the food or preferably in drinking water, tetracyclines in the water or by injection. Other water medications of value include erythromycin, sulphadiazine with trimethoprin.

Injection of penicillin and streptomycin simultaneously with vaccination has been successful in halting outbreaks of disease in turkey flocks. Food medication with tetracycline requires high levels of 300–400 g per ton over a prolonged period of 2–3 weeks for complete control and even then relapses are not uncommon.

On farms where there is a history of *P. multocida* infection then the use of a vaccine is recommended which can be obtained combined with *Erysipelothrix rhusiopathiae*. The first injection should be given at 7–8 weeks of age followed by a second injection four weeks later.

In the USA a live *P. multocida* vaccine is available in certain states. Administration is via the drinking water but can be associated with up to 4 per cent mortality. Inactivated adjuvented vaccines, in general, proved to be as efficacious.

MYCOPLASMOSIS

Avian mycoplasma have been implicated in several diseases in the turkey. The most important mycoplasma species involved in the turkey are *M. gallisepticum, M. meleagridis, M. synoviae* and *M. iowae*. The first two are not of major importance in commercial turkeys today as they have been eradicated in primary breeding stock and are therefore not transmitted to succeeding generations. However, some multi-age continuous production farms may still be infected.

The organisms are often found to be involved with other pathogens or predisposing factors such as viral or bacterial infections. Primary infection in the turkey is usually through the respiratory tract, the infected embryo or following artificial insemination.

Clinical signs associated with the disease may include coughing, sneezing, swollen sinuses and air sacculitis. Infections with both *M. gallisepticum* and *M. meleagridis* have also been associated with skeletal lesions, in particular a syndrome known as TS65 which involves the bowing of the legs in the region of the tarsus and metatarsus, frequently with swollen hock joints (Fig. 7.8).

Diagnosis on post mortem signs is not specific and isolation of the organism is the most certain method of confirming the diagnosis. On a flock basis the infection may be confirmed by demonstrating antibodies using rapid slide agglutination tests in the case of *M. gallisepticum, M. meleagridis* and *M. synoviae*. Serological tests on individual birds which are diseased are of little significance and should not be used in diagnosis as non-specific reactions caused by interfering factors are frequent.

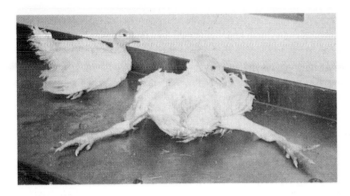

Fig. 7.8
Turkey with TS65 syndrome with splay leg and bowing of the legs in the metatarsal region.

Treatment can be carried out using a variety of drugs and antibiotics, such as tylosin, spectinomycin, erythromycin, lincomycin, tiamulin and the tetracyclines administered via the drinking water.

M. synoviae, although classically associated with joint lesions and synovitis, can be involved in mild respiratory signs or in association with viruses of Newcastle disease or avian influenza. *M. meleagridis* infection of turkeys has been associated with air sacculitis, abnormalities of the primary wing feathers in young poults, poor growth and chondrodystrophy. Clinical signs of chondrodystrophy reduced growth and wing feather abnormalities are symptomatic of TS65 and may occasionally be seen but differential diagnosis is essential for confirmation of *M. meleagridis* infection.

CHLAMYDIOSIS

Ornithosis, the disease in non-psittacine birds caused by *Chlamydia psittaci*, is not commonly diagnosed in turkeys in this country, but epidemics have occurred in turkey flocks in the USA, with sporadic outbreaks in the UK.

In the majority of flocks, signs are generally mild and may resemble other forms of respiratory disease with swollen sinuses and laboured breathing and greenish diarrhoea with blood may be present. Infection is usually by inhalation of infected material, following which the organisms multiply in the lungs and air sacs reaching kidneys, liver and spleen via the circulatory system.

On post mortem examination the lesions seen will depend upon the course of the disease. These include congestion of the lungs with fibrinous exudate in the pleural cavity, thickened air sacs and pericardial membrane and, frequently, a fibrin clot within the pericardial sac. Liver and spleen are generally enlarged and discoloured and may contain necrotic foci with a covering of fibropurulent exudate on the serosal surface.

Diagnosis can be based on post mortem examination of impression smears from liver or spleen for intracellular cytoplasmic inclusion bodies. Serological tests may be performed by specialist laboratories. Cultures should not normally be attempted due to the hazard presented to man, and material sent for laboratory diagnosis should be carefully wrapped before despatch. This disease is reportable in the UK.

Treatment with broad spectrum antibiotics is effective. Medication of turkeys with chlortetracycline in the food at a level of 200–400 g per ton for 3–4 weeks should suppress the clinical disease but does not necessarily eliminate the organisms completely. Initial treatment may be carried out via the drinking water at a concentration of 1–2 g per gallon.

ERYSIPELAS

Erysipelas is caused by *Erysipelothrix insidiosa* and is not uncommon in pole barn units on general farms in association with other diseases such as pasteurellosis. The source of infection is obscure. Sudden death in birds over 15 weeks of age is usually the first sign: occasionally younger birds are affected. Sometimes lethargy, head cyanosis and diarrhoea may be seen.

Post mortem findings are of generalized septicaemia with muscle and fat haemorrhages. The liver and spleen may be enlarged. Chronic cases may show signs of endocarditis. Confirmatory diagnosis depends on the isolation and identification of the organism. Blood smears may sometimes show Gram-positive rods.

Treatment of acute outbreaks is by injection of sodium crystalline penicillin and, or, long acting penicillin. Water and food medication is generally not very successful.

Prevention is by vaccination which can also be used in conjunction with treatment. Two doses of vaccine at intervals of four weeks is required for immunity; in fattening birds these would generally be given at 6 and 10 weeks of age.

SKELETAL DISORDERS

Diseases of the bones and joints are common in turkeys but rarely involve all the flock. Infectious conditions include osteomyelitis, bacterial synovitis, occasionally viral tenosynovitis or mycoplasma infections.

Uninfective conditions include rickets, tibial dyschondroplasia, twisted leg syndrome, crooked toes, rupture of the gastrocnemius tendon, splayed legs and abnormal gait.

Rickets may occasionally be seen in the young growing turkey of 2–6 weeks of age during the time of fast growth and mineralization of the bone. The turkeys requirement for vitamin D_3 is higher than the chicken and hence broiler or chicken diets should not be fed to turkeys at this age. Classic food deficiencies are unlikely in modern poultry diets. Where rickets is diagnosed, consideration should be given as to whether the food intake of the birds is satisfactory or to the possibility of another underlying disease such as chronic coccidiosis affecting food intake. The majority of birds in a flock will be affected and signs of a reluctance to rise and unsteady gait can be seen before development of bowing of the proximal tibia and sometimes an enlargement of the costochondral junctions and rib heads.

Diagnosis of rickets can be demonstrated on the finding of soft rubbery bones and beaks, and especially swollen rib junctions.

Rickets may be due to deficiencies of calcium, phosphorus, or vitamin D_3 or imbalances of the same. Mycotoxicosis may lead to poor absorption of vitamin D_3 or failure to convert in the liver to its active metabolites. Calcium deficiency or calcium phosphorus imbalances are extremely rare but it is important to remember that treatment of suspected phosphorus deficiency with vitamin D_3 preparations via the drinking water can exacerbate the condition by increasing calcium absorption. Treatment should be directed towards changing the feed if this is suspected as the cause. Subsequently feed should be sent for analysis for calcium, phosphorus and vitamin A levels, this being easily analysable in contrast to vitamin D_3 and acts as a marker for vitamin inclusion levels.

Mineral imbalances within subclinical rickets may in turn be involved in syndromes such as twisted leg and tibial dyschondroplasia where the aetiology of the condition is not clear. Twisted leg is characterized by lateral twisting and bending of the distal tibial tarsal and proximal tarsal and metatarsal bones. The condition is usually unilateral and sometimes associated with the gastrocnemius tendon slipping from the condyles.

Tibial dyschondroplasia is characterized by plugs of avascular and non-calcified cartilage in the metaphyses of the upper tibiotarsal and less commonly in the upper tarsometatarsal and tibiotarsal growth plate. Locomotor disturbance is frequently not observed in this condition which only becomes apparent at slaughter. On occasions birds will be observed with bowed legs and fractures of the tarsus. The incidence in flocks is generally of the order 2–3 per cent. Diets which induce metabolic acidosis increase the incidence of the disease and this may occur where excessive chloride is not balanced by extra sodium or potassium ions.

ACKNOWLEDGEMENTS

I gratefully acknowledge the assistance of J. C. Stuart in the compilation of this text and the provision of photographs.

REFERENCES AND FURTHER READING

Alexander, D. J. (1986) *Veterinary Record* **118**, 217.
Curtis, P. E. (1979) *Veterinary Record* **104**, 471.
Gordon, R. F. & Jordan, F. T. W. (1982) *Poultry Diseases*, 2nd edn. Edinburgh, Baillière Tindall.
Halrorson, D. A., Van Dijk, C. & Brown, P. (1982) *Avian Diseases* **26**, 634.
Hofstad, M. S. (1984) *Diseases of Poultry*. Ames, Iowa, Iowa State Press.
Joyner, L. P. (1978) *Avian Coccidiosis* (eds P. Long, K. N. Boorman and B. M. Freeman). Edinburgh, British Poultry Science.
McDougal, J. S. & Cook, J. K. A. (1986) *Veterinary Record* **118**, 206.

CHAPTER 8

Diseases of Game Birds

STEPHEN LISTER

INTRODUCTION

Game bird production in the UK has increased markedly in recent years. About 15 million birds are reared annually, mostly for sport, but also with some increased interest in table meat production. Conservative estimates suggest that it costs between £10 and £15 to put a bird in the air to shoot. However, the emergence of game shooting as a sport has meant that the high fees charged for a day's shooting have generated much interest in game rearing. Fees in excess of £15 per bird shot within a syndicate costing at least £2000 to join, confirm that the sport is now big business. Increased production has required the increased use of artificial incubation and custom hatching, increased number of birds placed under existing brooders and overcrowding in rearing pens. When this is combined with the fact that many enterprises recently set up may be managed by individuals previously unaccustomed to livestock production, there is obviously a need for considerable veterinary input.

Rearing units come in all shapes and sizes, and often veterinary advice is sought only on a "fire brigade" basis. The principal game birds likely to be presented to the general practitioner are the European pheasant (*Phasianus colchicus*), the common partridge (*Perdix perdix*) and the red legged or French partridge (*Alectoris rufa*). Most submissions will be pheasants and although the adults of these species present little problems in identification, their progeny are often virtually indistinguishable in their immature plumage, so good history taking may help avoid embarrassment!

GENERAL MANAGEMENT

Breeding hens may lay up to 50 eggs in a season lasting about 12 weeks between April and July, peaking in June. It is followed by intensive rearing up to eight weeks old. Hatchability of game bird eggs is generally very disappointing at about 65 per cent, compared with a figure usually in excess of 80 per cent for commercial poultry. With fertility estimated at about 90 per cent for game bird eggs, there is obviously considerable wastage of fertile eggs prior to hatching. Much of the wastage is related to management factors and the physical nature of the egg. Game bird eggs are laid directly into the environment and are usually faecally contaminated. The fact that the game bird egg shell is very thin leads to more cracks and makes bacterial penetration more likely. The egg is also more prone to excessive water loss by evaporation if storage conditions are poor. All these factors may lead to embryonic death or the production of small weakly poults.

Artificial incubation in hatchers is now the norm and the cost of incubation means that many smaller estates will send eggs away for so called "custom hatching". As a result, the sending away of dirty eggs together with poor hygienic conditions in hatchers can exacerbate the spread of egg-borne infections and introduce new agents to a premises with the return of the hatched poults.

Day-old poults are usually reared artificially in brooding pens ideally holding only about 100 poults/pen (Fig. 8.1). Unfortunately, production pressure usually demands groups larger than this and may lead to panic smothering or unevenness of growth. Birds are then moved into small rearing pens (Fig. 8.2) and then into release pens (Fig. 8.3) between six and eight weeks of age to acclimatize in an area close to where they will then be released into the wild.

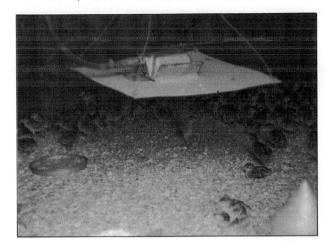

Fig. 8.1
Typical brooding pen.
Note food in shallow
open pans and overhead
heating.

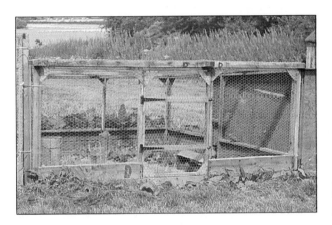

Fig. 8.2
Typical rearing pen
system.

DISEASE PROBLEMS (Table 8.1)

There are numerous disease conditions known to affect game birds and many of the infectious agents are those which afflict the commercial poultry industry. However, often the problems are either multifactorial or cannot be attributed to a specific disease agent.

Game bird rearing is very sensitive to management and husbandry practices because these birds are still essentially semi-wild rather than domesticated and also, due to a

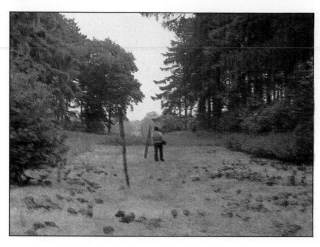

Fig. 8.3
Typical release pen close
to cover for eventual
release.

Table 8.1 Disease problems of game birds.

Management/nutrition	*Viral*
Starve outs	Marble spleen disease
Chilling	Rotavirus
Impactions	Newcastle disease
Navel ill	Infectious bronchitis
Rickets	Pox
Leg problems	ILT
Bacterial	*Mycoplasmas*
E. coli	M. gallisepticum
Salmonella species	M. columborale
Pasteurella species	M. synoviae
Staphylococcus species	M. gallinaceum
Erysipelas	*Fungal*
Mycobacterium species	Aspergillus
Yersinia species	Candida
Parasitic	*Intoxications*
Coccidia	Botulism
Syngamus species	Yew poisoning
Capillaria species	Pesticide misuse
Trichomonas species	Monensin toxicity
Hexamita species	*Others?*
Histomonas species	Turkey rhinotracheitis
Cryptosporidium	Swollen head
species	syndrome

historical lack of veterinary involvement, there is little appreciation of the basic rudiments of disease control.

In view of the influence of these management/husbandry factors on the manifestation of disease and attempted control, the more common disease conditions will be discussed in relation to the age of the bird affected. The areas to be considered will involve brooder (0–2 weeks old), rearer (2–8 weeks old) and release problems, the latter including consideration of problems in adult breeding birds.

BROODER PROBLEMS (0–2 WEEKS) (Table 8.2)

As indicated above, the semi-wild nature of game bird species can lead to problems with artificial brooding. While excessive light levels in pens may result in cannibalism, poults in low lighting may not find food and water with resulting deaths as "starve-outs". In this case, at necropsy, poults are small, the gizzard is empty with the lining being easily detached and the gall bladder is prominent confirming gut stasis. Panic smothering can occur in large groups, diagnosis usually being

Table 8.2 Age-related conditions affecting game birds.

Brooding period	Rearing period	Release/adult
"Starve outs"	Intestinal coccidiosis	Marble spleen disease
Smothering	Caecal coccidiosis	Syngamiasis
Chilling	Hexamitiasis	Yersiniasis
Impactions	Trichomoniasis	Avian tuberculosis
Cannibalism	Capillariasis	Coronavirus nephritis
Colibacillosis	Salmonellosis	Newcastle disease
Navel ill	Pasteurellosis	Infectious
Yolk sac infection	Erysipelas	laryngotracheitis
Renal failure	Yersiniasis	Infectious bronchitis
Aspergillosis	Syngamiasis	Swollen head syndrome
Rotaviral enteritis	Mycoplasma sinusitis	Poisoning
Salmonellosis	Rotaviral enteritis	
	Tail end syndrome	
	rickets	
	coligranulomata	
	non-specific enteritis	

made on farm by the distribution of deaths. Impactions of the proventriculus may occur, related to a combination of an immature digestive tract and poor presentation of food.

Infectious agents are usually only a problem at this age when precipitated by poor environmental conditions or management faults. As with commercial chicks, colibacillosis is often a reflection of poor chick quality or excessive environmental contamination, while aspergillosis usually indicates contamination in the hatchery or the use of mouldy bedding. In the latter, the post mortem picture is of small white smooth disc-like lesions up to 2 mm in diameter in air sacs or attached to the lung or dark nodules of varying size in the lung substance. Occasionally, torticollis and general imbalance can be caused by CNS fungal lesions, often visible to the naked eye as "space occupying lesions" of the cerebrum or cerebellum.

DULLNESS AND LETHARGY

A common syndrome in pheasant poults of less than 10 days old is a clinical picture of dullness and lethargy with drooped wings. Necropsy reveals a range of systemic disorders, usually presenting a fairly typical pattern of unhealed navels, yolk sac peritonitis, generalized septicaemia and renal failure. Mortality and morbidity can be very high with losses of 25 per cent of poults placed by 10 days of age being not uncommon, and this often leads to much argument/discussion between the rearer and the supplier of the day-old birds as to where the blame lies. Whereas obviously poor initial vigour and viability of day-olds may play a part, it is evident that the pressure to rear more birds per season has lead to far more poults being placed under existing brooder space. Where management and environmental control is less than excellent, problems are bound to arise. On some shoots there are reports of a good response to trimethoprim/sulphonamide water medication, but all too often by two weeks of age many birds will be half the weight of their contemporaries, barely having added to their original birth weight. In these cases it is usually advisable to segregate birds at this age according to weight, rearing on as several separate batches.

ROTAVIRAL ENTERITIS

A specific infectious agent causing early poult mortality and marked stunting and unevenness in brooding groups is rotaviral enteritis and this obviously needs to be considered when pictures such as that described above occur. In the case of rotaviral enteritis mortality rates of 70 per cent in the first week of life have been reported. Affected poults are very lethargic and dehydrated, but often do not show evidence of scouring. At necropsy, caeca are distended with copious frothy fluid usually ochre or beige in colour. There is often, also, thinning and ballooning of the intestinal wall generally along its length, the contents being clear and watery. This infection was first recognized and well documented as afflicting poults in the first week of life, but recent seasons have seen evidence of infection in age groups throughout rearing. This probably reflects the fact that this virus is now endemic in the environment and breeding stock in the UK, with maternal antibody protecting the younger age group. When such lesions are seen in poults over a week of age they obviously need to be differentiated from protozoal enteritis (see later), but suspicions should be aroused if this type of necropsy picture is associated with a failure to demonstrate the presence of protozoa in caecal and intestinal smears from freshly killed birds. Diagnosis at present requires the demonstration of rotavirus particles in intestinal contents by direct electron microscopy or polyacrylamide gel electrophoresis (PAGE).

REARING PROBLEMS (2–8 WEEKS) (Table 8.2)

In this age group the most common problems are related to intestinal parasites. Unfortunately an all too common diagnosis during this period is of "non-specific post-treatment enteritis". This syndrome usually arises when a keeper has already tried various stock treatments either as the wrong drug for the specific primary condition or the correct drug at the wrong concentration or for the wrong duration. As a result the initial precipitating agent is often masked by therapy or the group has reached a chronic "recovery" phase. Common sequelae in this "tail end" period are severe kidney damage (pale, swollen kidneys with excessive white urates in ureters), coligranulomata (irregular nodular swellings of the wall of the lower intestines and caeca), intestinal perforation and peritonitis or rickets resulting from prolonged malabsorption. A useful guide to adequate long bone mineralization is that by one week old well laid down bone should snap audibly when broken at necropsy. In these circumstances, satisfactory diagnosis, therapy and resolution can be a real headache.

If the practitioner is lucky enough to be called during the acute phase of an intestinal disorder at this age then prompt diagnosis and successful therapy is far more likely. As well as examining freshly dead carcases, at least six live ailing birds should also be requested, as accurate diagnosis of the motile intestinal parasites requires the examination of very fresh necropsy material.

COCCIDIOSIS AND SALMONELLOSIS

Coccidiosis remains all too common despite the presence of coccidiostats in most rations. There is field evidence of a lack of effectiveness of the widely used coccidiostat clopidol, but it is difficult to blame this solely on true drug resistance at a time when heavy stocking is causing increased weight of challenge on many shoots. There appears to be more evidence of a loss of efficacy of amprolium as a treatment in recent seasons. As a result of these factors, intestinal and caecal coccidiosis are still regularly diagnosed. Necropsy lesions cannot be described as consistent or pathognomonic. Indeed, the white cheesy caecal cores seen in caecal coccidiosis are similar to those of salmonellosis caused by *Salmonella binza* and *Salmonella derby* infection (Fig. 8.4). Diagnosis requires the examination of wet smears from the duodenum, several levels of the intestine and the caeca.

PARASITES

Mixed rotaviral and parasitic infections do appear to occur, making the examination of smears from freshly killed birds very important in aiding the diagnosis of infection with coccidia or the two motile protozoa *Hexamita meleagridis* and

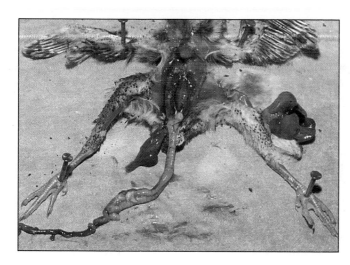

Fig. 8.4
Caecal salmonellosis.
Note white cheesy
caecal contents and
generally congested
carcase.

Trichomonas phasiani. Differentiation in smears is in the main achieved by experience, but as a general guide *Hexamita* is smaller showing jerky movement and a "flowing mane" under the light microscope or dark background illumination. *Trichomonas* species, on the other hand, are larger and pear-shaped having a slower motion with a discernible undulating membrane. Dimetridazole used to be considered effective against both agents but, more recently, appears less so specifically for trichomoniasis. High levels of tetracycline or furazolidone at the lower rate of 0.02 per cent have been suggested as alternatives.

Another intestinal parasite diagnosed in wet smears is *Capillaria.* The egg is usually a sandy brown colour with granular contents and has a distinct operculum at each pole. Often infestation with this fine worm (not usually visible with the naked eye in intestinal contents) causes clinical unthriftiness and weight loss rather than obvious enteritis and diarrhoea. Syngamiasis, caused by the gapeworm *Syngamus trachea*, can result in the sudden death of young poults caused by occlusion of the trachea by adult worms. Clinically affected birds demonstrate the typical clinical picture of "gapes" with repetitive mouth opening, pronounced respiratory effort and neck stretching, occasionally with blood present in the mouth. Adult worms can be seen easily in the tracheal lumen at necropsy (Fig. 8.5). Treatment with the fenbendazole

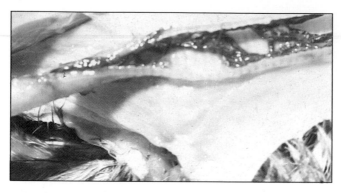

Fig. 8.5
Pheasant trachea
showing large
numbers of adult
Syngamus trachea
worms virtually
occluding the lumen.

mebendazole type of drugs can be effective but clinical relapse may occur where there are many immature worms and continued re-exposure, requiring a second treatment.

MYCOPLASMA INFECTION

A condition becoming more commonly diagnosed in recent seasons is infectious sinusitis associated with mycoplasma infection (Fig. 8.6). Initial presenting signs are varied; from sudden unexplained death to 100 per cent morbidity, affected birds showing inappetence, drooping wings, dyspnoea, and obvious "head cold" with head shaking, blepharospasm, keratitis, swollen infraorbital sinuses and rapid loss of condition. At necropsy, in the cases of sudden death, the findings can be very disappointing if only a cursory examination is made of the upper respiratory tract. In most cases the infraorbital sinuses at least show some slight

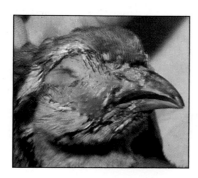

Fig. 8.6
Infectious sinusitis in a partridge.

swelling. Examination is easy either using the sharp end of the scalpel to slit the skin laterally beneath each eye or alternatively a transverse section of the beak just behind the external nares. This allows good visualization of the sinus contents. In the early stages, sinus and nasal turbinate mucus is copious and clear, later becoming thick and turbid, finally producing white caseous plugs in the sinus or hyperplastic areas around the external nares.

Laboratory examinations tend to show mixed overgrowths of *E. coli, Proteus* and *Pseudomonas* species by the time turbid material is present in the sinus. Selective cultures will yield mycoplasma (e.g. *M. gallisepticum, M. synoviae, M. columborale, M. gallinaceum*). Infection can arise anytime during the rearing phase but where breeding stocks are infected, the condition can arise in progeny during the first week of life. Response to therapy is usually very mixed, and probably reflects control of secondary infections rather than the precipitating mycoplasma. Tylosin and spiramycin are specific anti-mycoplasma drugs, but favourable results have been obtained with combined water medication with trimethoprim/sulphonamide, tylosin/sulphonamides, or dynamutilin at the pig concentration. Practitioners should be aware that dynamutilin can enhance the toxicity of any ionophore coccidiostats being used simultaneously. Affected birds are often reluctant to eat and drink so the introduction of additional drinkers during treatment may be beneficial. However, on some shoots, infection and disease can persist resulting in debility and emaciation of replacement breeding stock, and as with the situation in commercial poultry, the removal of this egg transmitted agent is virtually impossible without total depopulation.

Bacterial septicaemias can arise during the rearing phase, either as a complicating factor of some of the conditions described above or precipitated by sudden stresses or climatic changes. Septicaemic lesions due to *Pasteurella, Yersinia* and *Erysipelothrix* species need to be differentiated by cultural examinations, but are usually either self limiting or respond to tetracycline water medication.

RELEASE AND ADULT PROBLEMS (Table 8.2)

It is estimated that up to 20 per cent of pheasants die or leave the estate following release but before the shooting season commences and many carcases will not be located. Problems presented in this age group are often individual losses or related to trauma by prey or motor vehicle. However, birds on release and "free-ranging" breeder birds are prone to exposure to various toxic agents. These can include yew poisoning (notably ingestion of leaves in the autumn), lead poisoning where there is access to lead shot, avian botulism where the ingestion of only 1 g of toxin-carrying maggots may be lethal and pesticide intoxication where there is accidental or deliberate misuse.

In released birds, syngamiasis is usually associated with loss of body condition and sporadic deaths. Diagnosis often requires necropsy to demonstrate the reddish translucent adults in the trachea. Worms may be present only in the lower trachea close to the thoracic inlet requiring the whole length of the trachea to be examined as a routine. Other sporadic causes of loss of release birds include avian tuberculosis (Fig. 8.7) and yersiniasis, again diagnosis being fairly straightforward at necropsy.

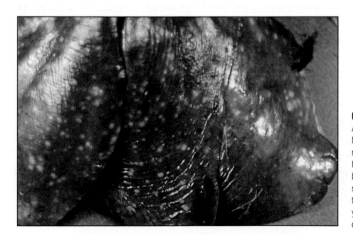

Fig. 8.7
Avian tuberculosis. Note widespread nodular lesions of the liver, spleen and bone marrow. Direct stained smears from these lesions would yield large numbers of acid-fast bacilli.

MARBLE SPLEEN DISEASE

One of the most consistent and frustrating conditions in pheasants in this age group is marble spleen disease, caused by avian adenovirus antigenically similar to that causing a haemorrhagic enteritis in turkeys. Characteristically very good condition birds die suddenly. The epidemiology and pathogenesis of this disease are not fully understood but it appears that infection is now endemic in the pheasant population, disease often being precipitated by some environmental factor. At necropsy, carcases are generally in excellent body condition and appear to have died from virtual drowning from acute lung oedema and congestion (Fig. 8.8). The spleen is enlarged and shows a characteristic mottling. Diagnosis is made by confirming the presence of the causal adenovirus in infected spleens by rapid agar gel precipitin test or characteristic intranuclear inclusion bodies similar to those of haemorrhagic enteritis in turkeys, histologically. Mortality may often persist for several days with the loss of good condition birds but unfortunately there is no specific treatment and ultimate control would depend on vaccination, although there is currently no licensed vaccine available in the UK.

VIRAL DISEASE

Virus diseases of game birds can occur following spread from domestic poultry. Pheasants are known to be very susceptible to Newcastle disease virus and the fact that the avian

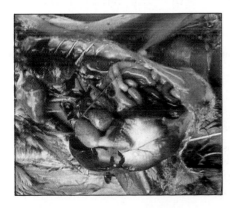

Fig. 8.8
Marble spleen disease. Note lung oedema and congestion, as well as enlarged mottled spleen.

paramyxovirus type I infection (a variant of Newcastle disease virus) is widespread in racing pigeons arouses at least the theoretical possibility of spread of infection to "free-range" game bird flocks. In a similar way infectious laryngotracheitis, avipox and infectious bronchitis virus infections have been recorded in game birds as a result of direct or indirect contact with domestic poultry or wild bird vectors.

Outbreaks of a syndrome very similar to that described as swollen head syndrome in commercial breeders and broilers have been reported in pheasants recently. It is known that pheasants infected experimentally with the pneumovirus associated with turkey rhinotracheitis and thought to be involved in swollen head syndrome, give a very good immune response and may show mild clinical respiratory disease. The role of these agents in game bird respiratory disease obviously warrants much further investigation.

CORONAVIRUS INFECTION

In recent seasons, a novel syndrome has arisen in adult pheasant related to infection with an, as yet, untyped coronavirus. The syndrome of coronavirus associated nephritis usually presents as sudden deaths of hens and cocks approaching full breeding condition or problems with egg production and mortality in hen birds in full production. At necropsy, there are widespread lesions of visceral gout and urolithiasis, very similar on gross pathology and histopathologically to that seen following infectious bronchitis virus infection (another unrelated coronavirus) in brown commercial egg layers. It seems likely that the virus causes kidney damage during rearing and the physiological stress approaching sexual maturity and a need to mobilize calcium for egg shell production precipitates terminal kidney failure. The result tends to be either a sudden outbreak of mortality at the beginning of the season or constant niggling losses throughout the season with some loss of egg size and colour. Attempted treatments seem fairly ineffective although supportive water soluble mineral/vitamin supplements are probably beneficial. The condition is distinct from the more common kidney damage seen in young rearing birds associated with water deprivation and climatic conditions or secondary to severe gut pathology.

CONCLUSIONS

Game birds present a varied and stimulating diagnostic challenge to the practitioner. The continued expansion of the industry has brought with it an increase in the severity of existing disease problems as well as some novel conditions. Increasingly practitioners will be met with requests for advice on parasite and disease control as well as the "fire-brigade" diagnosis of specific problems. Not only should the practitioner become conversant with the pathology and diagnosis of game bird diseases, but also the many aspects of husbandry and management that can have such a profound effect on the pattern of disease. Much advice and information is available through the Game Conservancy and there are still many lessons to be learnt from the commercial poultry industry.

There is considerable scope for client education on the need for prompt diagnosis in untreated birds at the first signs of trouble and the submission of suitable material for diagnosis, together with a more structured approach to parasite and disease control, hatching egg handling and flock management at the brooding, rearing and breeding levels.

FURTHER READING

Anon. (1987) *The Game Conservancy, Annual Review 1987*. Bridport Road, Dorchester, Friary Press.

Anon. (1987) *Some Diseases of Game Birds and Wildfowl*. Assorted booklets. The Game Conservancy Trust, Fordingbridge, Hampshire.

Gordon, R. F. & Jordan, F. T. W. (1982) *Poultry Diseases*, 2nd edn. London, Baillière Tindall.

Lister, S. A. (1989) *State Veterinary Journal* 43, 65.

Swarbrick, O. (1985) *Veterinary Record* 116, 610.

Partridge
  common, 116
  French, 116
Pasteurella spp., 125
Pasteurella multocida, 12–3, 32, 34–5,
    42–3, 47, 51, 53, 109–10
Pasteurella/Erysipelas vaccine, 92–3
Pasteurellosis, 18, 118–9
Peafowl, 69
Penicillin, 109, 112
Perdix perdix, see Partridge, common
Pericarditis, 20, 106
  serofibrinous, 19
Perihepatitis, 19–20, 106, 109
Permethrin, 82
Personnel: minimizing carriage of
    infection, 55
Pesticide poisoning, 118
Phasianus colchicus, see Pheasants
Pheasants, 71, 115 *and see* Gamebirds
Pigeons, 79, 81, 93
Piperazine, 12, 79
Poisoning, 30, 118–9
  botulism, 118, 126
  lead, 126
  monensin, 118
  nitrofuran, 100
  pesticide, 118
  yew, 118, 126
Poultry Meat Hygiene Regulations,
    17–8, 21, 26, 30
Poxyviridae, 41
Preventive medicine, 2–3, 54 ff
Processing of carcases, 25 ff
Proteus, 5, 97, 125
Pseudomonas spp., 97, 108, 125
Pyridones, 65

Quail, 69
Quinolones, 65

Râles, 33 ff
Red mite, 80–1, 84
Renal failure, 119
Reovirus, 32, 42, 44
Respiration, 3 ff, 31 ff, 97 ff
Rhinotracheitis,
  in gamebirds, 118
  turkey, 4–5, 7, 107–8, 118
Rickets, 113–4, 118–9, 122

Robenidine, 65
Rotaviral enteritis, 119, 121
Rotavirus, 6, 118–9
Rubbery beaks in turkeys, 113

Salinomycin, 12, 65, 102
Salmonella binza, 122
Salmonella derby, 122
Salmonella gallinorum, 29, 99
Salmonella pullorum, 28, 35, 99
Salmonella typhimurium, 99
Salmonellosis, 18, 28–9, 99 ff, 118–9, 122
Salphingitis, 23
Scaly beak mite, 82
Scaly leg mite, 82–3
Septicaemia, 18 ff, 97, 125
Sinusitis, 33, 45, 49, 110, 124
"Small round" virus, 61
Smothering, 119
Sneezing, 33 ff, 110
Spartakon, 79
Spectinomycin, 107
Spiromycin, 125
Splayed legs, 113
Spondylolisthesis, 10
Staphylococcus spp., 5, 12, 18, 24, 118
Starve out, 97, 118–9
Stocking densities, 15, 59
Streptococcus, 5
Streptomycin, 109
Stunning, 15
Stunting syndrome, 9
Sudden death syndrome, 10–1, 12, 112,
    124
Sulphadiazine, 109
Sulphamethazine, 109
Sulphaquinoxaline, 65, 102, 109
Sulphonamides, 64–5, 67
Swollen head syndrome, 118–9
Syngamiasis, 126
Syngamus trachea, 32, 44, 50–1, 53, 73 ff,
    79, 123–4
Synovitis, bacterial, 113

Tail end syndrome, 119
Tapeworms, 77–8
Tenosynovitis, viral, 113
Tetrachlorvinphos, 82
Tetracycline, 70, 106, 109, 123, 125
Tetrameres fissispina, 76–7

Index

Acidosis, 114,
Adenovirus, 32, 40, 42–3, 126
Air sacculitis, 18, 20–1, 110–1
Alcaligenes faecalis, 5, 106–7
Alcaligenes tracheitis, 106–7
Alectoris rufa, see Partridge, French
Amidostomum anseris, 77
Ammonia, 64
  excess, 32, 38 ff, 44, 46, 52
Amprolium, 64–5, 102, 122
Anaemia, 23
Anaticola, 84
Anorexia, 68, 109
Antibodies, maternal, 87
Arthritis, viral, 10
Arthropods, 73
Ascapilla, 79
Ascaridia spp., 75–6
Ascaris, 12
Ascites, 10–1, 14, 23, 30
Aspergillosis, 30, 97 ff, 118 ff
Aspergillus fumigatus, 21, 32, 34–5, 44–5,
    50, 53, 55
Avipox, 41

Blackhead, 27–8, 68–9
Bleeding of carcases, 27
Bordatella spp., 5, 107–8
Botulism, 118, 126
Breast blisters, 24
Bronchitis, infectious, 4, 6, 14, 32, 40,
    43–44, 47, 51–52, 90 ff, 118–9, 128
Brooder pneumonia, *see Aspergillus
  fumigatus*
Bruising to carcases, 26 ff
Budgerigars, 81–2

Bursitis, infectious, 88 *and see* Gumboro
  disease

Cachexia, 30
Calcium deficiency, 13–4
Cambendazole, 79
Canaries, 81
Candida, 118
Cannibalism, 14, 118
Capillaria spp., 12, 118, 123
Capillaria bursata, 75
Capillaria caudinflata, 75
Capillaria obsignata, 75
Carcase condemnation, 17 ff
Carcinoma, 22
Cardiohepatic syndrome, 100–1
  in turkeys, 14
Catena bacterium, 27
Ceratophyllus gallinae, 84
Cestodes, 77–8
Chlamydia psittaci, 111–2
Chlamydiosis, 111–2
Chlortetracycline, 106, 112
Citrazine, 79
Clopidol, 65, 67, 102
Clostridia, 97
Coal tar, 42
Coccidiosis, 6, 12, 59 ff, 66 ff, 91, 101 ff,
    113, 118–9, 122
Colisepticaemia, 39, 43, 51, 57, 105–6
Collibacillosis, 119–20
Conjunctivitis, 33, 45–6, 49, 69, 107
Contamination of carcases, 29–30
Control of Substances Hazardous to
    Health Regulations, 88–9
Coronaviridae, 40

Coronavirus nephritis, 119, 128
Coughing, 33 ff, 45, 69, 105, 108, 110
Crooked toes, 113
Cryptosporidium spp., 69–70, 118
Cyathostoma bronchialis, 73

Damage to carcases, 25 ff
Debeaking, 14
  turkeys, 96
Decoquinate, 65
Depluming itch mite, 82
Dermanyssus gallinae, 80–1
Diarrhoea, 5–6, 46, 48, 105, 109
  and see Faeces
  bloody, 104
Diazinon, 82
Dichlorvos, 82
Dimetridazole, 71, 103, 123
Ducks, 20 ff, 27, 67, 75–6, 84
Dynamutilin, 125
Dyschondroplasia, 9
  tibial, 113–4
Dyspnoea, 33 ff, 45, 47, 124

Egg drop syndrome, 6, 14, 91
Egg peritonitis, 12–3, 22
Egg production, 6 ff, 47
Eggs, shell-less, 46
Eimeria spp., 59 ff, 91, 101
Eimeria acervulina, 60, 62
Eimeria adenoides, 66, 101
Eimeria anseris, 67
Eimeria brunetti, 6, 60 ff
Eimeria colchici, 67
Eimeria duodenalis, 67
Eimeria maxima, 60 ff
Eimeria meleagridis, 66, 101
Eimeria meleagrimitis, 66, 101
Eimeria mitis, 60
Eimeria necatrix, 60–1
Eimeria nocens, 67
Eimeria phasiani, 67
Eimeria praecox, 60
Eimeria tenella, 60 ff
Eimeria truncata, 59, 67
Emaciation, 23, 25
Enteritis, non-specific, in gamebirds, 121
Enterococci, 97
Epidemic tremor, 7, 90–1

Erysipelas, 18, 112–3, 118–9
Erysipelothrix spp., 125
Erysipelothrix insidiosa, 112
Erysipelothrix rhusiopathae, 110
Erythromycin, 109
Escherichia coli, 4, 5, 18–9, 21, 24, 28, 32,
  36, 39, 42 ff, 49, 51, 53, 55, 97,
  105 ff, 118, 125
Ethopobate, 65, 102

Faeces
  sulphur-yellow, 68
  greenish, 111
  salmon pink, 60
  tarry, 105
Fenbendazole, 123
Fleas, 84
Flip over, 10–1
Formaldehyde, 2, 9, 55
Fowl cholera, *see Pasteurella multocida*
Fowl coryza, 32, 49
Fowl pox, 4, 32, 41, 43, 48, 52, 118
Furaltadone, 64, 99, 106
Furazolidone, 70, 99, 123

Gamebirds, 67 ff, 71, 74, 78, 115 ff
  hatching, 116
Gapes, 123–4, *and see Syngamus trachea*
Gapeworms, *see Syngamus trachea*
Gastrocnemius tendon, 113–4
Geese, 67, 73, 77, 84
Goniocotes, 84
Goniodes, 84
Gout, visceral, 8, 128
Green leg, 29
Guanidines, 65
Guinea fowl, 69
Gumboro disease, 88, 90 ff

Haemophilus paragallinarum, 32, 40 ff,
  45, 49, 53
Haemorrhagic enteritis, 6, 104–5
Halofuginone, 65, 102
Hatcheries, 55–6, 96–7
Hatching, gamebirds, 116
Head cold, 124
Heart failure, 10–1
Helminths, 73 ff
Herpesviridae, 40
Heterakis spp., 75 ff
Heterakis gallinarum, 69, 76, 103

Heterakis isolonche, 76
Hexamita meleagridis, 68–9, 122
Hexamitiasis, 70, 118–9
Histomongus meleagridis, 68–9
Histomoniasis, 27–8
  in gamebirds, 118
  in turkeys, 103
Hock joint, infection of, 12
Housing, 2, 54
  turkeys, 96
  ventilation, 3, 6
Hydropericardium, 21
Hygiene, 2–3, 8, 54 ff, 97
  meat hygiene, 17 ff

Influenza, 111
Influenza A, 20, 32, 42–3, 48, 52

Jaundice, 30

Kinky back, 10
Klebsiella, 5
Knemidocoptes, 81 ff

Lameness, 109
Laryngotracheitis, infectious, 4, 32 ff,
  40–1, 43, 45, 47, 52, 57, 118–9, 128
Lasalocid, 65, 102
Lead poisoning, 126
Leg disorders, 9–10
  of game birds, 118
Lesions
  larynx, 48
  liver, 27
  lung, 35–6
  skin, 25 ff
Leucosis, 22, 35
  lymphoid, 13
Levamisole, 79
Lice, 78–9, 84
Lipeurus, 84

Malathion, 82, 84
Marble spleen disease, 118, 127
Marek's disease, 13, 22, 25, 30, 35, 90 ff
Mebendazole, 79, 124
Mebenvet, 79
Mecanthus stramineus, 84
Menopon gallinae, 84
Methyl benzoquate, 65, 102
Methyl bromide, 64

Mites, 79 ff
Monensin, 65, 102
Monensin poisoning, 118
Moraxella, 5
Moraxella antipestifer, 107–8
Mortality, 8
  in turkey poults, 96
Mosquito bites, 41
Mycobacteria spp., 118
Mycoplasma columborale, 118, 125
Mycoplasma gallisepticum, 14, 32, 36,
  39 ff, 49, 51, 53, 110, 118, 125
Mycoplasma iowae, 110
Mycoplasma meleagridis, 14, 110–1
Mycoplasma synoviae, 14, 24, 32, 36,
  39–40, 43–4, 49, 51, 53, 110–1, 1
  125
Mycoplasmosis, 20, 34, 56–7, 110, 1
  124–5

Narasin, 12, 65, 102
Nasal exudate, 32, 49, 107–8
Navel ill, 118
Navel infection, 97, 118–9
Necrotic enteritis, 6
Nematodes, 44–5, 51, 73 ff
Neoplasms, 22–3
Nephropathy, 8
Newcastle disease, 4, 6–7, 14, 20, 3
  43–4, 46, 51–2, 57, 90 ff, 111, 1
  127–8
Nicarbazin, 65
Nilverm, 79
Nitrobenzamides, 65
Nitrofuran poisoning in turkeys, 1
Nitrofurans, 106
Northern fowl mite, 80–1

Oedema disease, *see* Cardiohepati
  syndrome
Omphalitis, 97
Ornithonyssus sylviarum, 80–1
Ornithosis, 20, 111
Osteomyelitis, 113
Overscald, 27
Oxytetracycline, 106

Paramyxovirus, 7–8, 39, 93, 128
Parasitism, 30, 44–5, 59 ff
Parrots, 79

Thiabendazole, 79

Tiamulin, 103

Torticollis, 109

Toxaemia, 97

Toxoplasmosis, 30

Trichomonads, 70–1

Trichomonas spp., 118

Trichomonas phasiani, 123

Trichostrongylus tenuis, 77

Trimethoprin/sulphonamide, 120, 125

Tuberculosis, 119, 126

Tumours, 30

  benign, 22–3

Turkey rhinotracheitis, 4–5, 7, 107, 118

Turkeys, 1, 4 ff, 7, 12, 14, 20 ff, 27, 68,
    81, 84, 87, 95

  cardiohepatic syndrome in, 14

  coccidosis in, 66 ff, 101 ff

Twisted leg, 9, 113–4

Tylosin, 125

Tyzzeria perniciosa, 67

Urolithiasis, 13, 12

Vaccination, 2, 52–3, 57, 87 ff

  in water, 89

  injection methods, 90

  spray, 89–90

  storage and disposal, 88–9

Valgus deformity, 9

Vitamin A deficiency, 32, 38–9, 41, 46,
    51–2

Vitamin D3, 113

Weight, 1

Welfare, 1 ff

Yersinia spp., 118–9, 125–6

Yew poisoning, 118, 126

Yolk sac infection, 97, 119